"Michael Tompkins has done a masterful job demystifying psychological problems, and illustrating how cognitive behavioral therapy (CBT) skills can be easily learned and applied to real-life situations. Readers gain a veritable treasure chest of tools to choose from, with step-by-step instructions for how to become proficient in utilizing the skills to improve coping, set meaningful goals, and change behavior to enhance quality of life. A must-have for anyone wishing to reduce emotional suffering."

—**Rochelle I. Frank, PhD**, assistant clinical professor of psychology at the University of California, Berkeley; and coauthor of *The Transdiagnostic Road Map to Case Formulation and Treatment Planning*

"This compendium of practical, specific tools guides readers through developing both *inside* skills—like how to think about thinking—and *outside* skills—like managing time and getting things done. With chapters on increasing your motivation and protecting your relationships with others, the guidance on offer is both specific and broad-based. Well organized—with clear rationales for each skill, and helpful worksheets—*The Cognitive Behavioral Therapy Workbook* is an excellent resource for both the general reader and for therapists."

—**Chad LeJeune, PhD**, founding fellow of the Academy of Cognitive and Behavioral Therapies, and author of *The Worry Trap* and *"Pure O" OCD*

"Life-changing. Keep this book near you and give it fifteen minutes of your attention every day. You will improve your well-being, your mood, and your productivity."

—**Jacqueline B. Persons, PhD**, director of the Oakland Cognitive Behavior Therapy Center; and clinical professor at the University of California, Berkeley

"This thoughtfully conceived and clearly written workbook, by a leader in the field of CBT, stands out as an excellent guide to strategies found to be most effective in producing significant psychological change. I firmly believe that this important book, which contains an array of helpful practice exercises, will be of great benefit to both readers looking for practical self-help tools and, also, to clinicians conducting therapy who can augment treatment with the material found in this valuable resource."

—**John Ludgate, PhD**, psychologist at CBT Counseling Centers in Western North Carolina, founding fellow of the Academy of Cognitive Therapy, and author of *CBT Resources for Therapists*

T0301213

"Tompkins is an internationally regarded clinician/teacher who shares his vast experience in a clear and appealing text. Readers who complete the book will learn important tools that will offer genuine life changes. For readers struggling with anxiety, depression, or other problems, the book will be highly valuable. The workbook identifies and explains the relationship between thoughts, feeling, actions, and attention. The chapters lead the reader to acquire a broad set of skills, ranging from mindfulness skills to thinking skills and interpersonal effectiveness skills. The chapters are well laid out and clearly delineate a program that offers the readers the opportunity to acquire a variety of core cognitive behavior skills to improve their lives."

—**Stuart Eisendrath, MD**, professor of psychiatry emeritus; and founder of the
UCSF Depression Center at the University of California, San Francisco

"*The Cognitive Behavioral Therapy Workbook* offers a practical guide for readers who want to take charge of their mental health. I appreciated the author's use of experiential learning throughout the book, as well as his knack for making complex concepts easily understood to appeal to a wide audience of readers. If you're looking for a down-to-earth, science-based mental health guide, this is a book you'll not regret purchasing!"

—**Joanne Chan, PsyD**, assistant professor of psychiatry at Oregon Health and
Science University, and coauthor of *ACT-Informed Exposure for Anxiety*

"With this book, Tompkins has authored a masterful application of self-help CBT, tied together neatly in a user-friendly package. His extensive training and wisdom grace every detail, from the strategic order of chapters to the clever exercises. This book wasn't written as a performative academic exercise—it's a genuine self-help tool sure to help countless readers. It's now at the top of my self-help recommendation list."

—**Gregory S. Chasson, PhD, ABPP**, licensed psychologist board certified in
behavioral/cognitive psychology, and associate professor in the department of
psychiatry and behavioral neuroscience at The University of Chicago

"This workbook is a must-have resource to update your mental health toolbox. Tompkins gives us a refreshing new take on the tried-and-true methods from CBT—which has a long track record of successfully helping people manage painful situations—by weaving in techniques from the fields of positive psychology and mindfulness practices. The user-friendly format makes it accessible to anyone who wants to boost their mental health self-care."

—**Valerie L. Gaus, PhD, ABPP**, psychologist in private practice, and author of
Cognitive-Behavioral Therapy for Adults with Autism Spectrum Disorder and *Living Well
on the Spectrum*

The
Cognitive
Behavioral
Therapy
Workbook

Evidence-Based CBT Skills to
Help You Manage Stress, Anxiety,
Depression, and More

MICHAEL A. TOMPKINS, PHD, ABPP

New Harbinger Publications, Inc.

Publisher's Note

NEW HARBINGER PUBLICATIONS is a registered trademark of New Harbinger Publications, Inc.

New Harbinger Publications is an employee-owned company.

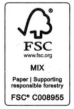

New Harbinger Publications, Inc.
5720 Shattuck Avenue
Oakland, CA 94609
www.newharbinger.com

Cover design by Sara Christian

Acquired by Jennye Garibaldi

Edited by Karen Levy

Library of Congress Cataloging-in-Publication Data on file

Printed in the United States of America

26   25   24

10   9   8   7   6   5   4   3   2   1   First Printing

For Lu, Mady, and Livie

Contents

Foreword

Cognitive behavior therapy (CBT) was developed by my father, Aaron T. Beck, MD, in the 1960s and 1970s. From its inception, CBT has included a strong therapeutic relationship, a cognitive case conceptualization, and a user-friendly skills-based approach to managing a variety of psychiatric, psychological, and medical problems as they arise in the here and now. At the Beck Institute for Cognitive Behavior Therapy in Philadelphia, the organization my dad and I founded, we have trained tens of thousands of clinicians from all over the world in this approach and continue our mission to improve lives worldwide through excellence and innovation in CBT.

The Cognitive Behavior Therapy Workbook is a great introduction to CBT and includes many of the skills we teach along with the core concepts and principles that make CBT one of the most commonly used psychological treatments in the world. In the workbook, you will find skills that you can use to quickly calm your mind and body as well as skills to change how you think about the events that trouble you. There are skills to manage time and tasks if you tend to procrastinate or want to improve your ability to get things done. Then there are skills to improve your relationships and decrease intense emotions, such as anxiety, depression, guilt, or shame. The workbook concludes with skills to enhance your life in positive ways.

You can use the workbook on your own or as a supplement to therapy or other treatments. You may want to suggest the book to friends and family members who are curious about CBT and explain how it might help you or them if they're struggling. Whatever challenges you face, you're likely to find skills that will help. I encourage you to read the book from start to finish and to practice each skill. Once you're familiar with all the skills, you'll likely return to the ones you find help you the most. Nearly a half century of research demonstrates that these skills help people feel better and live better and there's a good chance that they can help you, too. If you want to live with a greater sense of calm and well-being, I encourage you to read this workbook and learn and practice these skills.

—*Judith S. Beck, PhD*
President, Beck Institute for Cognitive Behavior Therapy
Clinical professor, University of Pennsylvania

Introduction

You are about to learn a set of powerful yet simple skills that have helped countless people around the world. These skills can decrease your anxiety, improve your mood, and help you accomplish more, get along with other people, and above all, live a fuller and more meaningful life. These are the skills you would learn in cognitive behavior therapy (CBT), a form of talk therapy that was developed by Dr. Aaron T. Beck in the 1960s.

CBT is a brief, structured, skill-based psychotherapy that has been scientifically tested and found to be effective in more than 2,000 studies for the treatment of many different health and mental health conditions (Butler, Chapman, Forman, and Beck 2006; Hofmann, Asnaani, Vonk, Sawyer, and Fang 2012).

The Cognitive Behavioral Model

CBT is based on the cognitive behavioral model of psychology, which assumes that it's not the things that trouble us but rather our view of those things that trouble us. By changing our thoughts, then, we can change the way we feel and act. The cognitive behavioral model includes the following:

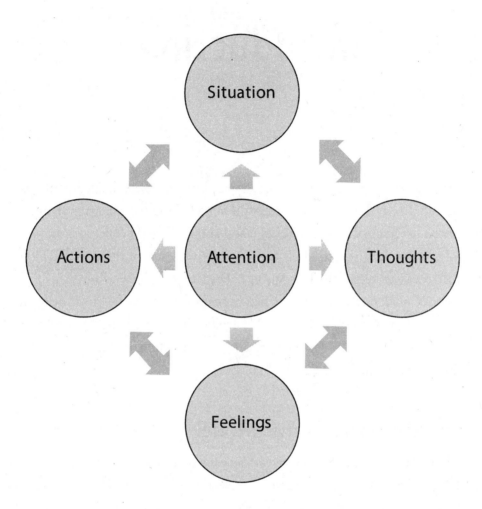

The Cognitive Behavioral Model

- **Thoughts:** Thoughts cause feelings. Our minds constantly generate thoughts and images. If you hear a sound in the dark and think, "That's someone breaking into the house," you might feel anxious. On the other hand, if you think, "That's the patter of rain on the window," you might feel relaxed and comfortable. The good news is that if you can change a thought, then you can change a feeling.

- **Feelings and physical sensations:** Feelings or emotions are part of our everyday life. There are positive feelings, such as joy, excitement, hopefulness, or serenity. There are negative feelings too, such as anger, anxiety, sadness, or guilt. Feelings include physical sensations or experiences, such as a racing heart or trembling hands. Feelings are signals. They alert us to possible danger. They orient us to a problem to solve. Feelings are perfect. If you feel anxious, you feel anxious. There is no debating a feeling. However, the thoughts that cause the feelings are open to examination and debate.

- **Actions:** Every emotion has a behavioral tendency or motivation. When you're anxious, you're motivated to be cautious and vigilant. When you're angry, you're motivated to strike out to defend yourself. When you're sad, you're motivated to slow down and seek solitude to regroup. There are "mental behaviors" too. These are thought actions, such as thinking through how to solve a problem or repeatedly thinking about a past hurt or slight. Thoughts can directly cause you to act too. For example, the thought, "I'll do it later," most likely means that you'll put off the task.

- **Attention:** Attention or awareness influence the other features of the model. When your attention rests on a feeling or physical sensation, the intensity of the feeling or sensation can increase in the way an itch intensifies in bed at night when you're less distracted and therefore more aware of the itch. When your attention goes to a thought, this awareness can increase the frequency of the thought. When your attention focuses on a behavior, this awareness can increase or decrease the frequency of the behavior.

The goal of CBT, then, is to learn skills to influence your attention, think reasonably about events and situations, and test out thoughts in the real world to see whether they're accurate or not. When you think more accurately or in more helpful ways, you'll feel better and be more willing to make small changes in your behavior. That's when things really start to change. Changing your behavior is the path to deep and lasting change. Changing your thinking is where you start.

The Workbook

This workbook includes a set of skills that you'll learn and then practice repeatedly, as problems arise, such as the abdominal breathing skill or the identifying thinking errors skill. These skills target the principle factors that experts believe maintain your emotional distress and interfere with living a full and successful life. There are many CBT skills, but there are two general types of skills that are likely to help most people with most problems:

- **Inside skills:** These CBT skills primarily target what's inside you: thoughts, attention, and the physical manifestations of feelings, such as tension and stress. Inside skills include skills to relax your body, change your thinking, and improve your ability to focus your attention.

- **Outside skills:** Not every problem is a problem with the way you think. There are real problems outside of you that are best managed with skills that can change the situation. Outside skills include skills to communicate clearly, prioritize and break down tasks, or schedule and plan ahead.

Some skills build on previous skills, so it helps to read through all the skill chapters from the beginning to the end the first time you use the workbook. You'll discover some skills work better for you than others. That's okay, but try all of the skills at least once, and then decide which ones are your go-to skills.

The workbook includes many examples that make each skill clear as well as worksheets and logs to help you to learn and practice the skills. Many of these materials as well as audio recordings of the meditations are available for download at the website for this workbook: http://www.newharbinger.com/52021. See the very back of this workbook for details.

In addition, the workbook includes experiential exercises to help you learn a skill from the inside out. Exercises might include questionnaires for you to complete, questions for you to answer, and activities for you to try that help you understand a skill and how it can help you feel better now.

In the final chapter, you'll learn to integrate all these skills into a plan to help you practice, and that's the rub. You're not likely to feel significantly better by just reading the workbook. Changing those unhelpful patterns of thinking and acting takes practice, but not as much practice as you might think. Just thirty minutes each day will help you feel better. Of course, you can practice more if you like. There's no downside to more practice. In fact, the more you practice, the more the skill becomes automatic. That's when you'll truly notice a change: with little effort, you'll automatically apply one of the many skills you've learned.

Now, take a moment and think about why you're reading this workbook. What do you want to change in your life? What do you do that you'd like to stop doing or do something more helpful instead? What are the ways you tend to think that cause you to feel needlessly anxious, or angry, or upset? How would you like to feel differently about yourself, about your future, or about the people in your life?

1. _____

2. _____

3. _____

The Audience

The audience for *The Cognitive Behavior Therapy Workbook* includes two groups. The first group includes people who are in CBT and would like a workbook to help them learn and practice CBT skills in their therapy. If you're already meeting with a therapist, take the workbook to your next therapy appointment so that you and your therapist can decide which skills would be particularly helpful in your therapeutic work together.

The second group includes people who are curious about CBT and want to learn CBT skills on their own. With diligence and practice, the skills in this workbook can help you achieve significant relief. However, if you're having a difficult time learning and practicing the skills, seek the services of a qualified cognitive behavior therapist.

The Path Forward

Perhaps you've tried other therapies or read other workbooks and you're feeling a bit hopeless that anything can help you live a more comfortable and fuller life. However, there's every reason to feel hopeful. The CBT skills in this workbook are powerful. Regardless of your genetics or the difficult moments you've experienced in your life, you can learn skills to manage your distress, improve your relationships, and, with time, transform your life.

You've likely heard the Chinese proverb, "A journey of a thousand miles begins with the first step." It reminds us of a basic truth about change: no matter how easy or difficult the change, the path forward begins with that first step or action. The path forward is reading the first page, practicing the first skill, and then the next and the next. That's the path forward: one small step at a time.

CHAPTER 1

Motivation Skills

Motivation is a willingness to start, continue, or stop a goal-oriented behavior (Wasserman and Wasserman 2020). In other words, motivation is the willingness to act in the direction of change. Motivation can change by the day and sometimes by the minute. Motivation is central to any behavioral change, whether it's increasing the frequency with which you exercise, eliminating after-dinner snacks, mastering your tennis backhand, or learning and practicing CBT skills.

Motivation skills are *inside skills* because they target the internal barriers to goal-oriented behavior: the thoughts and feelings that influence your willingness to act in the direction of change. An example is when it's time to practice a relaxation skill, such as progressive muscle relaxation, and you think, "I'm too busy right now. I'll do it later."

Why Are Motivation Skills Important?

The journey to deep and lasting change is neither easy nor straightforward. That's why skills to increase and maintain your motivation are essential. You'll use the motivation skills in this chapter in two ways:

- **To learn and practice skills:** Just like most skills you've learned in life—riding a bicycle, typing, or making friends—there will be moments when you wonder whether you can accomplish what you've set out to do. Learning and practicing the CBT skills in this workbook are not exceptions. Practice is the key and motivation is the skill that helps you practice and practice again.

- **To face uncomfortable feelings:** Perhaps there is no more difficult CBT skill to practice than the skill of facing (rather than avoiding) uncomfortable feelings or emotions. Whether your goal is to stand up for yourself, make more friends, or increase your energy, it's essential that you practice the skills you've learned when feeling uncomfortable or painful emotions. Motivation translates into willingness and willingness is the key to facing discomfort.

A Taste of Motivation

You've purchased this workbook and you're reading this chapter. That's a great first step. At the same time, although change begins with a first step, lasting change requires persistence, and persistence requires motivation. To get a taste of how difficult it can be to motivate yourself to do something, even if that something is easy, use the Taste of Motivation Log.

Instructions

1. To *get a taste of* motivation, set a goal for yourself to sit and do nothing for five minutes every day for one week. You're not to listen to music, scroll through your social media feeds, meditate, nothing. You're just to sit in silence with yourself.

2. Set a timer for five minutes. At the end of five minutes, record your experience on the Taste of Motivation Log. If you didn't do the exercise, record your experience on the log for that day too. Pay attention to *inside* barriers. These are the thoughts (for example, "I'll do it later" or "This is a waste of time") and feelings (for example, anxiety, irritation, or sadness) that arose that made it difficult for you to do the exercise that day. Perhaps *outside* barriers got in the way (for example, you couldn't find a quiet place to sit for five minutes, or you had a big project with a looming deadline).

Taste of Motivation Log			
Day	Time	Did you do it? (circle)	If you didn't do it, why not? What were the *inside* and *outside* barriers?
Sunday		Yes No	
Monday		Yes No	
Tuesday		Yes No	
Wednesday		Yes No	
Thursday		Yes No	
Friday		Yes No	
Saturday		Yes No	

Describe what you learned about your motivation. What were the inside and outside barriers to sitting for five minutes each day? Did anything surprise you in the exercise?

_____

_____

_____

_____

_____

_____

Skill: Set Goals

Setting goals is a motivation skill because, by definition, motivation focuses on increasing and maintaining goal-directed behavior. Just like entering the address of your destination in the GPS before you start a trip, clear goals describe the steps (left turn, right turn, straight ahead) you'll follow to get where you're going and how to tell when you've arrived. For example, if success means feeling less anxious, then what would you be doing differently? Would you speak more often to people you don't know well? Would you procrastinate less? If success means feeling less guilty, how would that present itself in your life? Would you more often say no to requests that you usually say yes to because you feel guilty saying no? Would you purchase fresh raspberries even when you feel guilty because you think it's such a splurge?

The best goals are specific and measurable (Doran 1981). Goals that are specific and measurable tell you where you're going, how to get there, and when you've arrived. A specific and measurable goal is usually a behavioral goal because the best measure of whether you've achieved a goal or not is to look at what you're doing or not doing. Here are some examples:

- Ask yourself: "What am I trying to accomplish or handle differently and in what specific situations?" "How would I like to act or behave differently?" For example, if your general goal is to be more assertive, your specific measurable goals might be, "Speak to my boss about a raise" or "Suggest a movie to my friend rather than waiting for her to decide."

- Ask yourself: "If I met my goal, what would I be doing differently?" or "How would I be reacting to situations differently?" For example, if your general goal is to improve your self-esteem, your specific measurable goal might be, "Sharing with my work colleagues what I accomplished this week" or "Dating people who are as successful as me."

- Ask yourself: "If I met my goal, what about my life would be different?" For example, if your general goal is to feel less depressed, your specific measurable goal might be, "Going out one weekend day per week with friends" or "Exercising for twenty minutes twice a week."

Look at the example worksheet and then set your own goals using the Specific and Measurable Goals Worksheet.

Instructions

1. Begin with a general goal, but rethink the general goal in terms of specific, measurable long-term, intermediate, and short-term goals. Remember to ask yourself the questions you've learned to help with this.

2. Describe a small step that you could take today to move closer to your goals.

Specific Measurable Goals

General Goal	Long-Term	Intermediate	Short-Term
Feel less irritated with my friends.	Don't blow up over little things my friends do or say.	Respond calmly and smile at the little things my friends say and do.	Leave the situation if I feel like I'm going to blow up.
Get along better with my spouse.	Go out with my spouse once each week and go away for the weekend once every three months.	Agree to watch a movie my spouse wants to watch and suggest short walks around the neighborhood with my spouse.	Don't blow up over little things my spouse forgets to do, like not closing the cabinet doors or not putting dirty dishes in the dishwasher.
Take better care of my health.	Do some form of aerobic exercise at least three times each week and eat healthy meals three times each day.	Lose six pounds this month.	Walk around the block every morning before work and on Saturdays ride my bike to and from the farmers market.
Be more assertive.	Express my preferences, limits, and opinions to friends, family, colleagues, and supervisor, comfortably and without qualification.	Say no to unreasonable requests from my supervisor (e.g., tell my supervisor to not call me on weekends or in the evenings).	Express my opinions to my friends.
Feel less anxious.	Do more activities on my own, feel less anxious speaking to people I don't know well, try new things with friends, volunteer to do things at work that I've never done before.	Say hello to strangers and don't check on my kids as much (e.g., no texts, don't call if they don't respond to my first text, don't repeatedly ask if they finished their homework).	Give presentations at work.
Increase my self-esteem.	Date people that I think are "a little out of my league," speak to my boss about a promotion, spend more time on weekends with friends.	Wear clothes that I like and express my preferences to my friends and family.	Accept compliments from others with a smile and a thank you.

Specific Measurable Goals						
General Goal						
Long-Term						
Intermediate						
Short-Term						

Skill: Consider the Costs vs. Benefits of Change

This is a simple skill that increases motivation through careful consideration of the costs and benefits of change versus the costs and benefits of staying the same. Motivation decreases when you focus too much on the reasons to stay the same. You might tell yourself that staying the same isn't so bad today because you're busy and can't spare ten minutes to practice a mindfulness skill. Or you might convince yourself that life is difficult enough, so why should you feel more uncomfortable by practicing one of the building emotion tolerance skills. You will consider the costs versus benefits in two separate steps.

Instructions

Look at the example worksheet and then choose a situation of your own to evaluate with the Look at Costs vs. Benefits of Change Worksheet.

1. Take a few minutes and think through all the costs and benefits of changing.

2. Do the same for staying the same. Be honest. You won't reach your goals by minimizing the costs of changing or by overemphasizing the benefits of staying the same.

Look at Costs vs. Benefits of Change Worksheet

Situation: Facing fear of panic attacks

	Costs	Benefits
Change	What if I have even more panic attacks? Maybe I'll find out that I'll never feel better. I barely have time to do my job. How will I do this too?	I won't worry so much about having a panic attack. I'll be able to keep my job and advance in my career. I'll feel better about myself if I overcome my worries.
No Change	My world will get smaller and smaller. I won't be able to move up in the firm because I'm too anxious. I'll become even more dependent on my partner, which stresses our relationship.	It's easier not to face my fear. Maybe I'm not cut out for my job. I could just quit and feel better immediately. Some days it's not so bad. Maybe this whole thing will go away on its own.

Look at Costs vs. Benefits of Change Worksheet		
Situation:		
	Costs	Benefits
Change		
No Change		

Take a Second Look at Costs vs. Benefits of Change

You may have focused on one side of the equation for so long—the costs of change or the benefits of staying the same—that you've developed tunnel vision and are overly focused on staying the same. The following skill can help you open your lens a little more so that change seems not only possible but desirable too. Examine the Look at Costs vs. Benefits of Change Worksheet you developed for a situation in the previous skill. Then take a second look at the costs versus benefits of change with the Take a Second Look at Costs vs. Benefits of Change Worksheet.

Instructions

1. Imagine that you invite a trusted friend or relative to provide the counterpoint to your points: the minuses of changing and the pluses of staying the same.

2. Imagine how they might challenge your assumptions in a noncritical and caring way and record their answers to the following questions:

   - What is a different view of this point?

   - Are there new opportunities you are missing?

   - Are there different possibilities that you could pursue?

   - Is there another way to look at this point that would increase your motivation?

   - Is there a way to change the minus of changing or the plus of staying the same in a way that encourages you to try?

Take a Second Look at Costs vs. Benefits of Change Worksheet

Situation: Facing fear of panic attacks

	Costs	Counterpoint
Change	What if I have even more panic attacks? Maybe I'll find out that I'll never feel better. I barely have time to do my job. How will I do this too?	Everything I've read about panic attacks tells me that if I practice some of the skills in this workbook, then I'm likely to have fewer panic attacks, not more. Even with the skills I've practiced so far, I'm already feeling a little better. Yes, my job is crazy, but life could get a lot easier if I practice the skills I've learned.
	Benefits	**Counterpoint**
No Change	It's easier not to face my fear. Maybe I'm not cut out for my job. I could just quit and feel better immediately. Some days it's not so bad. Maybe this whole thing will go away on its own.	Yes, it's easier to not face my fear, but my life is getting smaller and more difficult the longer this goes on. Quitting my job doesn't solve the problem. If I quit my job, I'd probably worry even more about money and finding another job. I've been struggling for months. I've cut back on my work. I've cut back on my stress level, but my anxiety is still really high. If it was going to go away on its own, it would have by now.

Take a Second Look at Costs vs. Benefits of Change Worksheet

Situation:

	Costs	Counterpoint
Change		

	Benefits	Counterpoint
No Change		

Skill: Consider the Concerns of Others

You likely have people in your life who love and care about you. They probably have told you that they're concerned about you and your struggles. Although it's essential that the motivation to change comes from within you, the concerns of others can encourage you to continue on your journey when your motivation dims. Record your answers on the Consider the Concerns of Others Worksheet.

Instructions

1. In the *Person* column, list the names of people in your life (friends, family members, colleagues, teachers, neighbors, faith leaders) who have voiced concerns about you and your struggles.

2. In the *Concern* column, list the specific reasons they shared with you. Try to be as specific as possible. It helps to translate concerns into behaviors, or what you're doing or not doing. For example, if the concern is "You're very depressed," list what the person observes when you're depressed (e.g., sleep most of the day, decline invitations to do fun activities).

3. In the *Reason* column, list the reasons for their concern. The reasons for their concerns include not only the effects they observe on you but also the effects they observe on themselves and others. For example, you might write in the *Reason* column the burden your spouse feels in taking care of the house and the kids because you put off doing things.

4. Reflect on each of the concerns and reasons. Ask yourself whether you can see their point of view, even a little. If you disagree with their concerns and reasons, consider what makes sense about their concerns, and why they might see this as a concern. Write this in the *Reason* column too. You may wish to review the worksheet with a trusted friend or family member and hear what they think about the concerns and reasons. Do they agree or disagree with the concerns? Do they have concerns of their own? Place this worksheet in a private place and read the list of *Concerns* and *Reasons* when your motivation wavers.

Consider the Concerns of Others Worksheet		
Person	Concern	Reason

Follow Your Values

You've learned to examine the costs and benefits of both changing and staying the same. Furthermore, you've learned to challenge the benefits of staying the same and developed a new point of view to help motivate you to change. However, you may require more to motivate you than these benefits and costs. You may require deeper reasons to change. Take a look now at another skill that can motivate you: follow your values.

Values are not the same as goals (Hayes, Strosahl, and Wilson 2016). Values are a direction or course (sailing south along the California coast) and goals are specific destinations or points (San Francisco, Santa Barbara, Los Angeles, San Diego) along the way as you move in the direction of a given value. Values are a process and goals are a product. For example, integrity is a value, and speaking truthfully and sensitively to colleagues and friends is a goal. Health is a value, and meeting yearly with your physician is a goal. Values aren't desires, wishes, or preferences, such as sex, money, or Indian food. Values are truths, beliefs, or understandings. Some values, such as charity or generosity, are in the service of others. Other values, such as creativity or spirituality, are most often in the service of your own welfare and growth. Values add meaning, purpose, and direction to our lives and thereby motivate us in deep ways. There are two steps to following your values:

1. Identify the values that will motivate you.

2. Develop value-action statements to motivate you.

Skill: Identify Your Values

Identifying core values is a process of reflection and discovery. Few of us take the time to identify what is truly important to us. This is not to say that your values aren't guiding and motivating you. If you're passionate about something, whether it's playing basketball or running for political office, a core value is likely leading the way.

Instructions

1. Read through the entire list of value words on the Identify Values Worksheet. As you read the value words, ask yourself:

    - What do I want to stand for when it comes to the value?

    - If I overheard people talking about what they admire about me, what words would I want to hear?

2. Next to each word, write a 1 2, or 3 (1 = most important 2 = important, and 3 = unimportant). Of these most important value words, select ten words. Then, from these ten words, select three to five of the most important value words. Write these words on the lines at the bottom of the worksheet.

Identify Values Worksheet		
Adventure	Excitement	Love
Autonomy	Fairness	Loyalty
Beauty	Family	Obedience
Challenge	Flexibility	Order
Clarity	Freedom	Originality
Cleverness	Friendship	Patience
Collaboration	Fulfillment	Peace
Commitment	Fun	Persistence
Communication	Happiness	Perspective
Community	Harmony	Power
Competence	Health	Prestige
Competition	Honesty	Productivity
Cooperation	Honor	Prosperity
Control	Humor	Purposefulness
Courage	Independence	Quality
Creativity	Influence	Recognition
Curiosity	Initiative	Relationships
Decisiveness	Innovation	Respect
Dependability	Integrity	Service
Diversity	Intelligence	Simplicity
Effectiveness	Intuition	Sincerity
Efficiency	Justice	Spirituality
Empathy	Kindness	Strength
Equality	Learning	Tolerance
Excellence	Legacy	Wisdom
_____	_____	_____

Now that you've identified three to five of the most important values, describe how well these values align with your actual behavior.

_____

_____

_____

_____

_____

_____

_____

Develop Value-Action Statements

In this next step, you'll develop value-action statements that you'll use to motivate yourself when your motivation dims. In other words, you'll translate values into action. Values in action are committed actions (Hayes et al. 2016). Committed actions include your willingness to consistently practice the skills in this workbook, as well as face discomfort, all in the service of your values. For example, if your value is integrity, then you'll tell the truth when a friend asks for your opinion, regardless of how worried you are that your friend may be upset with you. Or, if your value is relationships, then you'll face the discomfort of first dates and practice the communication skills in this workbook. Look at the example worksheet and then use the Develop Value-Action Statements Worksheet to develop a series of value-drive statements to motivate yourself at any time, but particularly when your motivation dims.

Instructions

1. Next to *Value Word*, write one of your three to five most important value words.

2. Next to *Value Action*, write a behavior or action that's consistent with and serves this value. Often this is the opposite of what you're avoiding doing or starting. For example, if you're avoiding practicing the relaxation skills in the workbook because you're too busy and can't find the time, then the opposite of this would be to practice a relaxation skill every day, regardless of how busy you are. Ask yourself, "What could I do that I'm not motivated to do?" Is it practicing a particular workbook skill? Is it practicing a skill when you're uncomfortable, such as assertively asking your boss for a raise, or doing some pleasant activities when you're depressed?

3. Next to *Value-Action Statement*, write one or two sentences that combine the value word and value action. Try to make the statement clear and powerful.

4. Before you practice a skill that makes you uncomfortable, or any time you notice that you're putting off practicing a skill or that you've lost your motivation to try, close your eyes and repeat the value-action statement to yourself several times. Imagine yourself doing the value action. Then, as you start the value action, repeat the value-action statement under your breath, as if you're talking yourself through it.

Develop Value-Action Statements Worksheet

Value Word	Integrity
Value Action	Express my opinions truthfully.
Value-Action Statement	In order to act with integrity, I will express my opinions truthfully to Gloria even though I'm worried that she'll think I'm stupid.
Value Word	Relationships
Value Action	Resolve conflicts.
Value-Action Statement	In order to strengthen and deepen my relationships, I will call Irma and apologize even though I'm worried that she'll be upset with me.
Value Word	Efficiency
Value Action	Send emails quickly.
Value-Action Statement	In order to act with efficiency, I'll read through emails only once and then send them even though I'm worried I've made a mistake.
Value Word	Learning
Value Action	Learn and practice relaxation skills in the workbook.
Value-Action Statement	In order to learn and improve my life, I'll practice two relaxation skills every day.

Develop Value-Action Statements Worksheet	
Value Word	
Value Action	
Value-Action Statement	
Value Word	
Value Action	
Value-Action Statement	
Value Word	
Value Action	
Value-Action Statement	
Value Word	
Value Action	
Value-Action Statement	

Skill: Rehearse in Your Mind

A simple way to increase your motivation to try something is to rehearse doing it first in your mind. It's also a great way to give yourself a practice run before you try a task. For example, say that you're planning to ask your boss for a raise and you're hesitating because you feel a bit nervous. Repeatedly rehearsing in your mind what you'll say will increase your confidence and thereby increase your motivation to try. In fact, you can rehearse in your mind first almost any skill in this workbook. For example, you might imagine going through the steps of solving a problem before you try it.

Instructions

1. Find a quiet place where no one will disturb you for ten minutes.

2. On a blank piece of paper, write the steps of the task you'll rehearse in your mind. For example, if the task is speaking to your boss about a raise, list all the steps in doing this. Include detailed sensory experiences in the steps you describe to make the scene feel more real. Imagine what you *see* around you (e.g., color of the walls, what people are wearing) and what sounds you *hear* (e.g., music, people's voices, or your voice as you speak). Feel the temperature on your skin. Do you feel cold or warm? The richer the scene you imagine, the more powerful the experience you create. Most importantly, describe applying the skill or completing the task successfully. For example, if the scene is to ask your boss for a raise, describe going through the assertiveness skill and then imagine that your boss says, "You deserve a raise. Let's talk about how big it will be."

3. Once you've written the scene, read through the script several times to familiarize yourself with it. Now, close your eyes and breathe slowly for one minute. When you're ready, rehearse in your mind the scene you've written. Remember to imagine that you successfully applied the skill.

Describe the effect on your motivation of rehearsing a skill in your mind before you try it for real.

_____

_____

_____

_____

_____

_____

_____

Skill: Take Another Seat

This is a powerful and fun skill to increase your motivation. The skill is based on the empty chair technique developed in psychodrama therapy (Moreno 2014). In a sense, you talk yourself into trying. Even if you don't try, you'll learn why you're not willing to try something that could help you feel and do better.

Instructions

1. Find a quiet room that has two chairs. Place the chairs across from each other. In your mind, label one chair the "Try" chair and the other the "Not Try" chair.

2. Sit in the "Not Try" chair. Imagine you're looking at your "Try" alter ego sitting in the "Try" chair in front of you. Now, talk to the "Try" alter ego and give all the reasons not to try. Don't hold back. Throw out every possible reason you can imagine to not try.

3. Now, move to the "Try" chair. Imagine you're looking at your "Not Try" alter ego sitting in the "Not Try" chair in front of you. Now, talk to the "Not Try" alter ego and give all the reasons you can imagine to try. Counter some of the reasons your "Not Try" alter ego gave for not trying.

4. Continue this for several minutes as you move from one chair to the other. Keep going until you've exhausted every conceivable reason that you can think of to try and to not try.

5. Now, on a blank sheet of paper, write all the great reasons you came up with to try and the counterpoints to the reasons you came up with to not try.

Describe the effect on your motivation of the Take Another Seat skill.

_____

_____

_____

_____

_____

_____

_____

_____

Wrap Up

Like any skill, particularly those that are new and sometimes difficult to learn and practice, persistence and willingness are the keys to deep and lasting change. The motivation skills in this chapter will help you learn and practice the other workbook skills, but you'll go back to these skills over and over when your motivation dips and your willingness falters. You'll find this to be particularly true when you practice the emotion exposure skills later in the workbook. Facing uncomfortable feelings is a challenging skill to master. Maintaining your motivation through the process is critical.

In the next chapter, you'll learn skills to dampen the physical tension and arousal that accompany emotions, particularly anxiety, anger, and sadness. The CBT skills we'll cover are a great place to start. They're easy to learn and apply and can help you feel better immediately.

CHAPTER 2

Relaxation Skills

Whether you're feeling anxious, angry, guilty, or ashamed, your body is likely tense. Relaxation skills are *inside skills* because they target the physical manifestation of these emotions. Relaxation skills are a great introduction to the power of CBT because they're easy to learn and practice and can provide you with some immediate relief. You may have learned relaxation skills on your own and already know firsthand how helpful they can be when you want to calm your emotional system. There are many relaxation skills that are used in CBT. In this chapter, you'll learn two basic types:

- **Breathing skills:** This set of relaxation skills targets the depth and rate of your breathing. Breathing skills are a powerful way to quickly and easily calm your body and mind and thereby dampen your emotional reactions to events.

- **Muscle relaxation skills:** This set of relaxation skills targets muscle tension. Muscle relaxation skills are an effective way to reset your arousal system, and daily practice can inoculate you against the buildup of excessive stress throughout the day.

Although the relaxation skills in this chapter focus on calming your emotional system by controlling your breath and relaxing your muscles, *attention* plays a role in calming your emotional system too. That's because these relaxation skills include a present-moment anchor for your attention. In abdominal breathing, you observe the feeling of the breath in the moment, or focus on repeating a word or phrase. In progressive muscle relaxation, you observe the feeling of tensing and then relaxing each muscle group in the present moment. In visualization relaxation, you focus your attention on an image in the present moment. Learning to direct your attention to the present moment is a powerful technique to calm both your body and your mind. In the next chapter (Chapter 3: Mindfulness Skills), you'll learn other skills to harness the power of attention in calming your emotional system.

Why Are Relaxation Skills Important?

Relaxation skills are important for three reasons:

- **A tense body tends to intensify emotions, such as anger, anxiety, or shame.** Perhaps you've noticed that when you're feeling physically tense, you're more irritable and less patient. A tense body sets you up to react more intensely to life events. Relaxation skills decrease physical arousal and tension and thereby decrease the frequency and intensity of your emotional reactions.

- **A tense body tends to increase the frequency of unhelpful thoughts.** For example, the longer you worry, the more difficult it is to stop. That's because physical tension increases the activity of your mind: more tension, more thoughts. Soon you're in an escalating cycle of thoughts, physical tension, more thoughts, more physical tension. Relaxation skills calm the body and mind, which interrupts this cycle.

- **The more anxious, angry, or sad you feel, the more strongly you believe the situation (or your read on the situation) is true.** This is called emotional reasoning. For example, if you feel guilty about something, you may believe that the guilty feeling "proves" that you've done something wrong. Any objective evidence that you haven't done anything wrong is ignored or dismissed in favor of the assumed "truth" of the feeling. Relaxation skills dampen your emotional reaction to events and once you're feeling calmer, it's easier for you to step back and see what is true rather than what "feels" true.

The goal of relaxation skills, like any skill in this workbook, is to build your capacity to move automatically and without much thinking into a relaxed state or attitude. It's the way repeated practice of a physical skill builds "muscle memory." Muscle memory enables you to quickly and automatically catch a pass or hit the correct piano key.

How Do Relaxation Skills Work?

Your nervous system is composed of two parts. The *central nervous system* (CNS) controls most functions of your body and mind. The CNS includes the brain and spinal cord. The *peripheral nervous system* (PNS) includes two main parts: the somatic and autonomic nervous systems. The somatic nervous system enables you to move your muscles and relays information from your ears, nose, and eyes to your brain. The *autonomic nervous system* (ANS) controls involuntary bodily functions, such as your heart rate, breathing rate, and digestion.

The ANS is composed of two parts or branches: the sympathetic branch and the parasympathetic branch. The sympathetic branch activates the stress response. Body tension is part of the stress response, along with increased heart rate and blood pressure, slowed digestive functioning, increased blood flow to the extremities, and increased release of hormones like adrenaline to prepare your body to protect itself from a perceived threat or difficult situation. The parasympathetic branch opposes the sympathetic branch and activates the relaxation response.

Relaxation skills target the parasympathetic branch of the ANS. The relaxation response restores your body to a calm state when the stress response is triggered. Simply put, the relaxation response is the opposite of your body's stress response—your "off switch" to your body's tendency toward stress. Relaxation skills are a powerful way to move your body toward a state of physiological relaxation, where blood pressure, heart rate, digestive functioning, and hormonal levels return to normal.

Controlled Breathing Skills

Breathing is fundamental to life and a sensitive index of your emotional state. The rate and depth of your breathing reflect the state of your emotional system as well as regulates it. The goal of breathing skills is to regulate the depth and pace at which you breathe. Regulating your breath calms your nervous system (McCaul, Solomon, and Holmes 1979; Clark and Hirschman 1990). Most people aren't conscious of the way they're breathing but, generally, there are two types of breathing patterns:

- **Chest (thoracic) breathing:** This type of breathing comes from the chest and involves short, rapid breaths. You likely breathe this way when you're feeling stressed, anxious, angry, or upset. You may not even be aware that you're breathing this way when you're upset. Chest breathing can disrupt the oxygen and carbon dioxide exchange and thereby decrease the concentration of oxygen in the blood. A lower level of dissolved oxygen in your blood results in a number of uncomfortable physical sensations (for example, dizziness, nausea, sweating) and can amplify your general physical and emotional discomfort.

- **Abdominal (diaphragmatic) breathing:** This type of breathing is deep, even breathing that engages your diaphragm, allowing your lungs to expand and creating negative pressure that drives air in through the nose and mouth, filling your lungs. This is the way newborn babies naturally breathe. You're also probably using this pattern of breathing when you're in a relaxed stage of sleep. Abdominal breathing stimulates the parasympathetic nervous system (relaxation response), which calms your emotional system.

Caution: The following breathing skills are safe for most people. However, if you have a medical condition, such as asthma, chronic obstructive pulmonary disease (COPD), or other lung or heart concerns, talk with your doctor before starting the practice.

Skill: Breathe with Your Abdomen

Abdominal or diaphragmatic breathing is a simple way to regulate the depth and rate of breathing. As you become more comfortable with abdominal breathing lying down, try it sitting up and then standing up. With practice, you'll be able to shift into abdominal breathing throughout the day whether you're sitting at your desk or standing in line at the grocery store.

Instructions

1. Lie on your back with your knees slightly bent and your head on a pillow. You may place a pillow under your knees for support.

2. Place one hand on your upper chest and one hand below your rib cage on your abdomen. Notice how your abdomen rises with each breath in and falls with each breath out. If you wish, replace the hand on your abdomen with a book and place your hands at your sides.

3. Now, imagine that a long tube runs from your nose to a balloon in your abdomen. Slowly inhale through your nose, feeling your abdomen rise beneath your hand. If it's difficult for you to feel your abdomen rising and falling, lie on your stomach and rest your head on your folded hands. Inhale deeply so that you can feel your abdomen push against the floor.

4. Once you know what it feels like to breath diaphragmatically, slow and deepen your breath. Inhale slowly through your nose and exhale slowly through pursed lips as though you're breathing through a straw.

5. Focus on the slow rise and fall of your abdomen. When your attention swings away from your breathing to thoughts, feelings, or physical sensations, just notice them and return your attention to your breathing.

6. At the end of each abdominal breathing practice, notice and enjoy how you feel for one minute.

7. Practice abdominal breathing for five minutes, once or twice a day. Gradually extend the time you practice to twenty minutes, twice a day.

Skill: Breathe Four Square

Four-square breathing, also known as box breathing, is very simple to learn and practice. In fact, if you've ever noticed yourself inhaling and exhaling to the rhythm of a song, you're already familiar with this type of paced breathing.

Instructions

1. *Inhale* through your nose as you count to four.

2. *Hold* the air in your lungs as you count to four.

3. *Exhale* through your nose as you count to four.

4. *Hold* your lungs empty as you count to four.

5. *Inhale* through your nose as you count to four.

6. *Hold* the air in your lungs as you count to four.

7. *Exhale* through your nose as you count to four.

8. *Hold* your lungs empty as you count to four.

9. Repeat the pattern for up to ten minutes.

10. Take a few additional minutes and focus on how your body feels.

Skill: Breathe 4-7-8

The 4-7-8 breathing skill acts as a natural tranquilizer for the nervous system. Paced breathing such as this is the most effective breathing method to improve mood and decrease physiologic arousal (Balban et al. 2023). The held breath (for seven seconds) is the most critical part of this practice. This pause allows oxygen to re-saturate your bloodstream. However, the absolute time you spend on each phase is not as important as the ratio of 4:7:8. If you have trouble holding your breath for seven seconds, shorten the length that you hold your breath, but keep to the ratio of 4:7:8 for the three phases. With practice, you can slow your breathing to match the 4:7:8 ratio more closely.

Instructions

1. Find a place to sit or lie down comfortably. Rest the tip of your tongue against the roof of your mouth, against the ridge of tissue behind your upper front teeth. Keep your tongue in place throughout the practice.

2. Inhale quietly through your nose as you count four to yourself.

3. Hold your breath as you count seven to yourself.

4. Exhale through your mouth, around your tongue, making a whoosh sound as you count eight to yourself.

5. Practice this pattern for four cycles.

Muscle Relaxation Skills

Edmund Jacobson was an American physician who in the 1930s proposed that a relaxed body is incompatible with uncomfortable feelings, such as anxiety, stress, or anger (Jacobson 1938). Muscle relaxation skills involve learning to discriminate when your muscles are tense and when they're relaxed and how to release that tension quickly and effectively.

Skill: Relax Your Muscles Progressively

Relaxing your muscles progressively, also known as progressive muscle relaxation (PMR), is an exercise that relaxes your mind and body in two steps:

1. Apply muscle tension to a specific part of the body. This step is essentially the same regardless of which muscle group you target. First, focus on the target muscle group, for example, your left hand. Next, take a slow, deep breath and squeeze the muscles as hard as you can for about five seconds. In this instance, you'd make a tight fist with your left hand. It's important to *really feel* the tension in the muscles, which may even cause a bit of discomfort or shaking. It's easy to accidentally tense other surrounding muscles (for example, the shoulder or arm), but try to tense only the specific muscles you target. Isolating muscle groups gets easier with practice.

2. Quickly release the tensed muscles. After about five seconds, let all the tightness flow out of the tensed muscles. Exhale as you do this step. You will feel the muscles become loose and limp as the tension flows out. *It's important to deliberately focus on and notice the difference between the tension and relaxation. This is an important part of the skill.* It takes time to learn to relax the body and to discriminate between tension and relaxation. At first, it may feel uncomfortable to be focusing on your body, but with time, it can become quite enjoyable. Remain in this relaxed state for about fifteen seconds, then move on to the next muscle group. Repeat the tension-relaxation steps. After completing all of the muscle groups, take some time to enjoy the deep state of relaxation.

Progressive muscle relaxation can focus on four, eight, twelve, or sixteen muscle groups. The following progressive muscle relaxation emphasizes sixteen muscle groups. If you feel any pain or discomfort when tensing any muscle group, feel free to omit that step. To increase the relaxed state, visualize your muscles tensing and a wave of relaxation flowing over them as you release that tension.

Number	Muscle Groups	
4	Face	Abdomen and chest
	Arms, shoulders, and neck	Lower limbs (feet and legs)
6	Face	Abdomen
	Both arms	Chest by deep breath
	Shoulders and neck	Both lower limbs (feet and legs)
8	Both arms	Shoulders
	Both lower limbs (feet and legs)	Back of neck
	Abdomen	Eyes
	Chest by deep breath	Forehead
12	Lower arms	Shoulders and lower neck
	Upper arms	Back of neck
	Lower legs and feet	Lips
	Thighs	Eyes
	Abdomen	Lower forehead
	Chest by deep breath	Upper forehead
16	Lower arms	Shoulders, Lower neck
	Upper arms	Back of neck
	Legs	Lips
	Feet	Eyes
	Thighs	Lower forehead
	Abdomen	Upper forehead
	Chest by deep breath	

Instructions

1. Begin by finding a comfortable position either sitting or lying down in a location where you will not be interrupted. Allow your attention to focus only on your body. If you begin to notice your mind wandering, bring it back to the muscle group you're working on.

2. Take a deep breath through your abdomen, hold for a few seconds, and exhale slowly. Again, as you breathe, notice your stomach rising and your lungs filling with air.

3. Tighten the muscles in your forehead by raising your eyebrows as high as you can. Hold the tension as you count five to yourself. Now, abruptly release the feeling of tension. Pause as you count ten to yourself.

4. Now smile widely, feeling your mouth and cheeks tense. Hold the tension as you count five to yourself, and then release. Appreciate the softness in your face. Pause as you count ten to yourself.

5. Next, tighten your eye muscles by squinting your eyelids tightly shut. Hold the tension as you count five to yourself, and then release. Pause as you count ten to yourself.

6. Gently pull your head back as if to look at the ceiling. Hold the tension as you count five to yourself, and release, feeling the tension melt away. Pause as you count ten to yourself. Feel the weight of your relaxed head and neck. Breathe in and breathe out. In and out. Let go of all tension, stress, and discomfort.

7. Tightly but without straining, clench your fists. Hold this position as you count five to yourself, and then release. Pause as you count ten to yourself.

8. Now flex your biceps. Feel that buildup of tension. Visualize the biceps tightening. Hold this position as you count five to yourself, and then release. Pause as you count ten to yourself. Enjoy the feeling of limpness. Breathe in and breathe out.

9. Now tighten your triceps by extending your arms and locking your elbows. Hold this position as you count five to yourself, and then release. Pause as you count ten to yourself.

10. Now lift your shoulders as if they could touch your ears. Hold this position as you count five to yourself, and then quickly release, feeling their heaviness. Pause as you count ten to yourself.

11. Tense your upper back by pulling your shoulders back, trying to make your shoulder blades touch. Hold this position as you count five to yourself, and then release. Pause as you count ten to yourself.

12. Tighten your chest by inhaling deeply. Hold this position as you count five to yourself, and then slowly exhale all the tension. Pause as you count ten to yourself.

13. Now tighten the muscles in your stomach by sucking in. Hold this position as you count five to yourself, and then release. Pause as you count ten to yourself.

14. Tighten your buttocks. Hold this position as you count five to yourself, and then release. Imagine your hips falling loose. Pause as you count ten to yourself.

15. Tighten your thighs by pressing your knees together as if you were holding a penny between them. Hold this position as you count five to yourself, and then release. Pause as you count ten to yourself.

16. Now flex your feet, pulling your toes toward you and feeling the tension in your calves. Hold this position as you count five to yourself, and then release. Feel the weight of your legs sinking down. Pause as you count ten to yourself.

17. Curl your toes under to tense your feet. Hold this position as you count five to yourself, and then release. Pause as you count ten to yourself.

18. Now imagine a wave of relaxation slowly spreading through your body beginning at your head and going all the way down to your feet. Feel the weight of your relaxed body. Breathe in and breathe out as you enjoy the warm, relaxed feeling in your body.

Skill: Release-Only to Relax

Once you've learned to discriminate between a tense versus a relaxed body through progressive muscle relaxation, you can shorten the time it takes to relax your muscles with the release-only variation, which removes the tension step in progressive muscle relaxation. For example, instead of tensing your stomach and chest before relaxing them, you move directly to relaxing the muscles. At first, the feeling of relaxation can feel less intense than when you tensed the muscles beforehand, but with practice, the release-only technique can feel just as relaxing.

The release-only skill works best after you've practiced progressive muscle relaxation with sixteen muscle groups for a few weeks, then one or two weeks with twelve muscle groups, then one or two weeks with six muscle groups, and finally several weeks with four muscle groups. Feel free to progress through the four groups as slowly or as quickly as you like, as long as you've mastered a muscle group before moving on to the next muscle group. The following instructions for the release-only skill include the four group progressive muscle relaxation: 1) face; 2) arms, shoulders, and neck; 3) stomach and chest; and 4) lower limbs (legs and feet)

Instructions

1. Take a deep breath through your abdomen, hold for a few seconds, and exhale slowly. As you breathe, notice your stomach rising and your lungs filling with air.

2. Imagine warmth and relaxation flowing into your face as you say "release" to yourself. Pause as you count ten to yourself.

3. Imagine warmth and relaxation flowing into your arms, shoulders, and neck as you say "release" to yourself. Pause as you count ten to yourself.

4. Imagine warmth and relaxation flowing into your stomach and chest as you say "release" to yourself. Pause as you count ten to yourself.

5. Imagine warmth and relaxation flowing into your legs and feet as you say "release" to yourself. Pause as you count ten to yourself.

Skill: Relax on Cue

The relax-on-cue skill, also known as cue-controlled relaxation, decreases the time it takes to relax your body to one or two minutes. The goal of cue-controlled relaxation is to build a link between the relaxation response and a cue word or phrase, such as "breathe in" or "let go." In this way, you relax your body quickly as you say the cue word to yourself. Cue-controlled relaxation builds on the release-only progressive muscle relaxation you learned earlier, so make sure you're comfortable and confident with release-only relaxation before practicing the cue-controlled relaxation skill.

Instructions

1. In a location where you will not be interrupted, sit comfortably in a chair with your hands in your lap, palms up, and your feet flat on the floor. Take a deep breath through your abdomen, hold for a few seconds, and exhale slowly. As you exhale, imagine blowing the tension of the day away slowly. Empty your lungs as you feel your abdomen and chest relax.

2. Now, using the release-only relaxation skill, quickly relax each of the four muscle groups: face; arms, shoulders, and neck; stomach and chest; and legs and feet. Try to relax completely in thirty seconds or less, if you can.

3. Continue to breathe deeply and slowly. As you inhale, say "breathe in" to yourself. As you exhale, say "let go" to yourself.

   Breathe in... Let go...

   Breathe in... Let go...

   Breathe in... Let go...

   With each breath in, inhale feelings of peace, comfort, and calm. With each breath out, exhale tension, discomfort, and stress. Feel at ease now as your abdomen and chest gently move in and out with slow, relaxing breaths. With each breath, the feeling of relaxation deepens and spreads across your body.

4. Continue this way for several minutes, repeating to yourself "breathe in" and "let go" while you breathe comfortably. Focus your attention on these words as the words form in your mind and then fade away. Feel your muscles relax more and more with each slow regular breath.

5. Continue to breathe deeply and slowly as you say "breathe in" and "let go" to yourself.

   Breathe in... Let go...

   Breathe in... Let go...

   Breathe in... Let go...

6. Continue to breathe as you say these words to yourself for several more minutes. Feel each breath in bring calm, comfort, and peace. With each breath out, feel tension, discomfort, and stress float away. After ten or twenty minutes, and if you have time, repeat the cue-controlled relaxation skill.

7. Practice cue-controlled relaxation twice each day. Because the goal of cue-controlled relaxation is to learn to relax quickly, pay attention to the time it takes to deeply and completely relax.

Quick Relaxation Skills

Sometimes you don't have ten minutes to breathe or thirty minutes to relax your muscles. You want to relax quickly in the moment. Here are several relaxation skills that activate your relaxation response quickly and easily.

Skill: Apply Relaxation in the Moment

The applying rapid relaxation in the moment skill is just what it sounds like: relaxing quickly when in an anxiety-evoking or stressful moment (Öst 1987). This skill builds on skills you've already learned and practiced: progressive muscle relaxation, release-only relaxation, and cue-controlled relaxation.

By now, you're likely very aware of signs that your body is tense. It's important to know these first signs of physical tension, along with other signs of intense stress or upset (for example, rapid breathing, sweating, rapid heartbeat, trembling, nausea, or light-headedness), in order to apply this skill quickly to short-circuit the stress response before it builds. As soon as you notice any sign of stress, follow these three steps.

Instructions

1. Take two or three slow, deep breaths.

2. Say these calming words (or the relaxation word or phrase with which you've practiced) to yourself as you continue to breathe slowly and deeply:

   Breathe in… Let go…

   Breathe in… Let go…

   Breathe in… Let go…

3. Scan your body for tension and relax the muscles you don't require to continue your activity. For example, as you sit at your computer to respond to a stressful email from a coworker, relax the muscles in your chest, abdomen, and buttocks while your shoulders, arms, and hands remain active as you type.

Skill: Release Tension Quickly

This quick relaxation skill combines releasing muscle tension and visualization. With practice, you'll bring on the relaxation response in a few seconds just by imagining squeezing the toothpaste or lemon and then spreading open your hands.

Instructions

1. Grab two tennis balls, one in each hand. If you don't have tennis balls, use balled-up washcloths or socks.

2. Close your eyes and squeeze the tennis balls as you imagine squeezing toothpaste out of a tube or juice out of a lemon. Squeeze as you count to five, then release as you spread open your hands.

3. Squeeze again as you count to five, then release as you spread open your hands. Repeat three times.

Skill: Relax and Refresh

As one stressful day leads to another, it may feel like you're walking through a fog of intense emotion. Try this simple quick relaxation skill to climb out of that emotional fog and see things as they really are.

Instructions

1. Sit in a comfortable chair and close your eyes.

2. Imagine your stress is like a dense, heavy fog that's swirling around you. Take several deep breaths as you imagine standing and walking up a hill.

3. With each step, softly say "relax and refresh" to yourself as you walk up the hill and the fog thins.

4. Continue to imagine walking up the hill as the fog becomes thinner and thinner until you reach the top of the hill.

5. Now, take a moment and look around. Below you is the fog of stress, churning and swirling. Before you are majestic mountaintops, a bright blue sky, and a beautiful valley spreading out before you as far as you can see.

6. Take several deep breaths as you softly say "relax and refresh" to yourself. Finish by resting several minutes above the hustle and bustle of stress at your feet.

Wrap Up

Relaxation skills are powerful strategies to calm your body and mind and are easy to learn and practice. Just ten or twenty minutes per day at least once or twice a week can make a big difference in how you feel. In addition, some of these calm body skills work great in the moment when you're feeling distressed and want to reset your emotional system quickly.

In the next chapter, you'll learn simple skills to harness the power of your attention. The mind and body are connected: Tense mind, tense body. Tense body, tense mind. Mindfulness skills are a powerful way to feel better in the moment and from one moment to the next.

CHAPTER 3

Mindfulness Skills

Mindfulness is the act of being fully aware—of whatever is happening inside and outside of you—in the present moment without judging or criticizing your experience or yourself. Mindfulness has been a feature of many religions for thousands of years, from Buddhism to Hinduism, as well as in Christianism, Islam, and Judaism (Trousselard, Steiler, Claverie, and Canini 2014). More recently, mindfulness as a secular practice has emerged in the West, although even the Western tradition of mindfulness rests upon the foundation of Eastern religions and traditions (Kabat-Zinn 1982; 1990). Mindfulness as practiced in the West includes:

- **Intention to cultivate awareness of the present moment (and return to it again and again).** Mindfulness is the act of choosing to attend to one thing and not to another. Although immersion in the present moment can occur spontaneously, such as when you're engrossed in drawing something, mindfulness as a skill requires you to actively and repeatedly choose to direct and redirect your attention to the present moment.

- **Observing rather than reacting to what is occurring in the present moment.** We tend to pull away from what we dislike. Therefore, it's essential that you cultivate a nonjudgmental, curious, kind, and accepting attitude toward yourself and your experience in order to rest fully in the present moment. If you're judging yourself or your experience, then you're not paying attention to what's happening in the moment. If you're criticizing yourself about a mistake you made two weeks ago in a presentation to your work team, or worrying about making the same mistake next week when you present to the team again, then you're not focusing on what's happening now. Instead, you're living in a painful past or an anxious future.

Mindfulness skills are *inside skills* because they target the internal experiences—your thoughts, physical sensations, and actions—through the act of repeatedly directing attention to these experiences as they arise in the present moment and without judging or criticizing yourself or your experiences.

Why Are Mindfulness Skills Important?

Studies show that practicing mindfulness skills, even for just a few weeks, can bring a variety of physical, psychological, and social benefits. For example, mindfulness skills alone or in combination with other psychological interventions can decrease stress, anxiety, and other negative emotions (Chambers et al. 2008; Hofmann, Sawyer, Witt, and Oh 2010). For example, mindfulness skills can augment the effectiveness of other skills you'll learn in this workbook, such as emotion exposure skills and emotional well-being life skills.

Experience Mindfulness

Mindfulness sounds mysterious to some people, but it's not. You've likely experienced mindfulness but didn't know it. For example, when you've ordered a meal at an expensive restaurant, you likely paid attention to the meal in a way that you don't pay attention to your cereal in the morning. With an expensive meal, you might take a moment to look at the way the food is arranged on the plate and the color of the foods. You might take a moment to inhale the aroma of the food and feel the warm, delicious smells circle your face. When you taste the food, you intensely attend to the flavors and the feel of the food in your mouth. That's mindful eating. In this exercise, you'll practice eating a raisin—although any food will do—with that same intention.

Instructions

Go to a quiet room where you won't be disturbed. Turn off your phone and sit in a comfortable chair. Read the following instructions and, if you like, record and then listen to it. During the skill, focus your attention on each aspect of the experience in the present moment (hold, see, touch, smell, listen, place, taste, swallow, follow).

1. **Hold:** Pick up the raisin and place it in the palm of your hand or between your finger and thumb. Focus on the raisin and imagine that you've come to Earth from a distant planet and you've never seen an object like this before. Study the weight and feel of the raisin in your hand. As you explore the raisin, move the raisin around in your palm or between your fingers.

2. **See:** Look at the raisin. Bring your full attention to the raisin as you explore every part of it with your eyes. Notice the folds and where the light shines. Notice the darker hollows, the folds and ridges, and any asymmetries or unique features. Notice the color and the breaks in the skin of the raisin and any sugar crystals on the surface of it.

3. **Touch:** Touch the raisin and turn it over between your fingers. Explore its texture, perhaps with your eyes closed if that enhances your sense of touch. Feel any softness, hardness, coarseness, or smoothness as you softly touch the raisin.

4. **Smell:** Hold the raisin beneath your nose. Inhale the fragrance of the raisin. With each inhalation, take in any smell, aroma, or fragrance that may arise. As you inhale, notice anything interesting that may be happening in your mouth or stomach.

5. **Listen:** Bring the raisin close to your ear. Now, squeeze it and roll it between your fingers. Listen for any sound. Do you hear a pop, a squish, or a rustle?

6. **Place:** Now slowly bring the raisin to your lips. Notice how your hand and arm know exactly how and where to position it. Perhaps you become aware that your mouth waters. Gently place the raisin in your mouth. Let it rest on your tongue without biting it. Spend a few moments and explore the raisin with your tongue. Notice the sensations of having the raisin in your mouth. Gently move the raisin around in your mouth. Notice the movement of your tongue and jaws.

7. **Taste:** When you are ready, bite down on the raisin. Notice how and where it needs to be in your mouth to chew it. Then, very consciously, take one or two bites of the raisin. Notice any waves of taste. Now chew the raisin and notice the saliva in your mouth and how the texture of the raisin changes as you chew. Without swallowing yet, notice the sensations of taste and texture in your mouth and how these may change over time, moment by moment.

8. **Swallow:** When you feel ready to swallow the raisin, notice the sensations as you prepare to swallow the raisin. Now, swallow the raisin. Notice the sensations as it moves to the back of your tongue and down your throat.

9. **Follow:** Finally, notice the feel of the raisin as it moves down into your esophagus and on its way to your stomach. Take a moment to sense how your body as a whole feels after completing this exercise.

As you practiced mindfully eating a raisin, you may have noticed your mind wander away from the experience of eating a raisin in the present moment. That's okay. In fact, that's normal and natural. Our minds naturally distract us from the present moment. When you recognize that your attention has drifted away from the present moment, acknowledge that your attention has wandered and gently return your attention to the present moment anchor. In this case, the present moment anchor was the multitude of experiences (smell, sight, taste, touch) that you observed fully as you mindfully ate a raisin.

Describe what you noticed (sight, smell, sound, taste, and touch) while eating the raisin (or other food). What thoughts, memories, or images arose? Did anything surprise you in the exercise?

_____

_____

_____

_____

_____

_____

_____

Types of Mindfulness Skills

There are two types of mindfulness skills in this workbook:

- **Formal skills:** Formal mindfulness skills build a consistent and regular practice. Without a formal practice, the benefits of mindfulness are not sustainable over time.

- **Informal skills:** Informal mindfulness skills integrate a mindful attitude into everyday activities, such as walking or eating, to generalize the benefits of mindfulness into life.

Formal Mindfulness Practice

In a sense, the goal of a formal mindfulness practice is to build your mind's capacity to shift into a mindful attitude quickly and without much effort. Most mindfulness experts will tell you that at least thirty minutes per day of mindfulness practice is necessary to build this capacity. It's not necessary to practice thirty minutes from the start. You can build up to thirty minutes in steps, perhaps five minutes at a time. However, the most important element to build a mindful capacity is to practice every day.

To build a formal mindfulness practice, practice the next two mindfulness skills (body scan and the ring of light) three times a day. Start with just two minutes of practice each time and add a minute as you become more comfortable and confident up to five minutes. Once you reach five minutes per practice, try bundling these five-minute practices into a single fifteen-minute practice. Once you're comfortable with one fifteen-minute practice per day, add five minutes each week until your daily practice is thirty minutes. The benefits of these longer periods of mindfulness practice can last for many hours, which makes it well worth the time you set aside to do it. To help you remember to practice, link it to something you do every day. For example, before you shower, before you eat, before you brush your teeth, or before you go to bed.

Skill: Scan Your Body

A body scan is the foundation of a *formal* mindfulness practice because it's easy to learn and apply. A body scan involves systematically moving your attention from one part of your body to the next, usually moving from the feet to the top of the head, noting any physical sensations, such as tingling, tightness, warmth, or even the absence of sensations.

It's best to do the body scan lying down on the floor or on a soft surface, but if you can't lie down, do the body scan while sitting in a comfortable chair. Read aloud and record the following script and listen to it.

Instructions

As you are lying on whatever surface you're on, notice what it feels like to be lying there. Noticing the sensations present in this moment, noticing temperature, noticing points of contact with the body and the surface, noticing the rise and the fall of the abdomen. Allowing the body to rest in this position and noticing sensations as you breathe in and as you breathe out.

Feeling the air move in and out of your body, let's begin by bringing attention to the toes of your left foot. With the in-breath, noticing the sensations present or lack of sensation. And then with an out-breath, let go of the toes and move your attention to the bottom of the left foot, including the heel touching the floor. Noticing all the sensations present in that region of the body, also notice how lack of sensation is something the mind can be aware of. Move on to the top of your left foot and ankle, noticing sensations present or lack of sensation. Now move into the lower leg, knee, thigh, and hip on the left side of the body.

Moving awareness, now, to the toes of the right foot, the bottom of the right foot, including the heel touching the floor. Bringing awareness to the sensations present in that part of the body. Moving on to the top of your right foot and ankle and scanning that region with awareness, noticing sensations present or lack of sensation. Now move into the lower leg, knee, thigh, and hip on the right side of the body.

Bringing awareness now to the pelvic region, noticing sensations present or lack of sensation.

Bringing awareness to the lower back and abdomen, aware of what's there, without judgment or assessment, simply noticing with awareness.

Continuing to scan the back, rib cage, and chest.

Moving now to the shoulder blades and shoulders, noticing what is present in those regions of the body.

From here, go to the fingers and the hands, the left and right together. Tuning into the fingers, thumbs, palms, and back of the hands, noticing what's there, noticing sensations present in the hands and the fingers.

Now moving awareness to the wrists, forearms, elbows, upper arms, and shoulders, and noticing what sensations are present in those regions of the body. On an out-breath, let go of the whole of the arms and the hands.

Moving now to the neck and the throat, noticing what is there or not there.

Moving on to the head and face, and scanning with awareness the jaw, chin, lips, teeth, gums, roof of the mouth, tongue, the back of the throat, cheeks, and nose. Feeling the air moving in and out of the nose. Then bringing awareness to the ears, eyes, eyelids, eyebrows, forehead, temples, and scalp, holding the whole of that region with awareness.

Now stay in the present moment with the breath flowing in and out of the body, simply awake to whatever arises and predominates in your field of awareness at any given moment. And this may include thoughts or feelings, sensations, sounds, the breath, stillness, and silence. Be with whatever comes up in the same way you were with the scan.

Notice how you may tend to react to impulses, thoughts, memories, and worries. Let yourself purposefully observe them without rejecting or pursuing. Practice simply seeing and letting go, seeing and letting go. No agenda other than to be present and awake.

Coming back into the room, fully awake and fully present. As we bring this practice to a close, may we be peaceful and at ease, may our hearts be soft and open, may we be safe and protected, and may our bodies be healthy and strong.

Skill: Sit in the Ring of Light

The ring of light is another *formal* mindfulness practice skill. The ring of light mindfulness skill primarily targets the physical sensations in your body, and if you're a visual person, the ring of light might work better for you than the body scan.

Before you practice this skill, read the instructions to familiarize yourself with the skill and then keep the instructions nearby in case you wish to refer to them as you practice. Alternatively, read aloud and record the following script and listen to it.

Instructions

Take a few slow, deep breaths as you close your eyes. As you continue to breathe, imagine a narrow ring of light that circles the top of your head like a halo. Imagine the light glows an intense color—white, blue, green, yellow—whatever color feels comfortable and interesting.

As you continue to breathe with your eyes closed, notice any physical sensations where the light touches. Perhaps you'll notice your scalp tingling or itching. Perhaps you'll notice a warm feeling on your forehead or above your ears. Whatever sensations you notice are okay.

Now, imagine the ring of light slowly descending around your head, passing over the tops of your ears, your eyes, and the bridge of your nose. As the ring descends, become aware of any sensations you feel, even small sensations. Notice any muscle tension or discomfort you may feel on the top of your head and forehead.

Imagine the ring of light continuing to descend over your nose, mouth, and chin. Observe any physical sensations you may notice where the ring of light illuminates.

Continue to imagine the ring of light descending around your neck and notice any feelings on your throat or the back of your neck and where your neck touches your shoulders.

Now imagine the ring of light widening as it moves down your torso, across the tops of your shoulders, and across your biceps. Notice any sensations, muscle tension, tingling, discomfort, or pleasant feelings that you might feel in your shoulders, upper back, and upper arms.

As you continue to breathe slowly and deeply, imagine the ring of light descending around your arms and toward your hands. Notice any feelings or sensations where the light touches on your upper arms, elbows, forearms, wrists, hands, and fingers. Become aware of any tingling, itching, or discomfort you might hold in these places.

Now become aware of the light touching your chest, the middle of your back, the sides of your torso, your lower back, and stomach. Notice any discomfort or tension that you feel in those places, no matter how small they might be.

As the ring of light continues to move down toward your feet, become aware of any sensations you feel in your pelvis, buttocks, and upper legs. Notice any feelings in the fronts and backs of your legs. Continue to watch the ring of light slowly descend around your lower legs, around your calves, shins, feet, and toes. Notice any discomfort or tension you feel in these places.

Notice the ring of light grow fainter around your feet and then disappear. Continue to take a few slow, deep breaths. When you feel comfortable and ready, open your eyes and return your attention to the room.

Informal Mindfulness Practice

The goal of *informal* mindfulness skills is to integrate a mindful attitude into everyday activities. Unlike a formal practice that you do every day for a set period of time, you apply informal mindfulness practice briefly but frequently throughout the day. In this way, informal mindfulness practice is spontaneous, flexible, and woven into the fabric of each and every day. Applying mindfulness skills to moments in your life not only creates calm moments but also enhances the pleasure and meaning of life itself. You'll learn three simple informal mindfulness skills: breathe mindfully, focus on a single object, and act mindfully.

Skill: Breathe Mindfully

This informal mindfulness skill is about anchoring to the present moment and there may be no better anchor to the present moment than the breath. No matter where you go, there you are and there it is. Practice mindful breathing for a few minutes while you walk, or at the end of your lunch, or during a work meeting, or while watching television. The more you pair mindfulness to the activities in your life, the more you'll remember to take a mindful attitude to them.

Before you practice this skill, read the instructions to familiarize yourself with the skill and then keep the instructions nearby in case you wish to refer to the instructions as you practice. Alternatively, read aloud and record the following script and listen to it.

Instructions

Close your eyes or fix your eyes on a spot in front of you and bring your attention to your breathing. Observe your breathing as if you've never encountered breathing before. Observe your breathing as if you're a curious scientist who wishes to observe the process closely without judgment. Notice the air as it comes in your nostrils and down to the bottom of your lungs, and notice the air come back out again. Notice how the air is slightly cooler as it goes in and slightly warmer as it goes out.

Notice the gentle rise and fall of your shoulders with each breath [pause for five seconds] *and the slow rise and fall of your rib cage* [pause for five seconds] *and the comfortable rise and fall of your abdomen* [pause for five seconds]. *Rest your attention on one of these areas now, whichever you prefer, on the breath moving in and out of your nostrils, or on the gentle rise and fall of your shoulders, or on the easy rise and fall of your abdomen. Rest your attention on this spot and notice the in and out of the breath.*

Whatever feelings, urges, or sensations arise, whether pleasant or unpleasant, gently acknowledge them, as if nodding your head at someone passing by on the street, and return your attention to the breath. [Pause for ten seconds.] *Whatever thoughts, images, or memories arise, whether comfortable or uncomfortable, gently acknowledge them and let them be. Let them come and go as they please and return your attention to the breath.*

From time to time, your attention will wander away from the breath, and each time this happens, notice what distracted you and then bring your attention back to the breath. No matter how often you drift off into your thoughts, whether a hundred times or a thousand, simply note what distracted you and return your attention to the breath. [Pause for ten seconds.] Again and again, your mind will wander away from the breath. This is normal and natural and happens to everyone. Our minds naturally distract us from what we're doing, so each time this happens, gently acknowledge it, notice what distracted you, and then return your attention to the breath.

If frustration, boredom, anxiety, or other feelings arise, simply acknowledge them, and return your attention to the breath. [Pause for ten seconds.] No matter how often your mind wanders, gently acknowledge it, note what distracted you, and return your attention to the breath.

Skill: Focus on a Single Object

This *informal* mindfulness skill is a great way to practice mindfulness in stressful situations, such as in a meeting or in a difficult conversation with a friend. During stressful or difficult situations, your mind is particularly prone to take you away from the present moment, as it wanders from one thought to another, because the present moment is where you're feeling anxious, frustrated, or guilty. At these times, you might focus on the button on the shirt of the person speaking to you or on the pattern of his tie. It doesn't matter what it is as long as you can see it while you continue to listen and reply to the person.

As with any mindfulness skill, you'll become distracted by your thoughts, physical sensations, and the sights, sounds, or smells in your environment. That's okay. As long as you acknowledge that your attention has wandered and gently and kindly return your attention to the single object, you're doing great. Locking your attention on a single object and keeping it there isn't possible, and even if it were, that's not mindfulness.

Before you practice this skill, read the instructions to familiarize yourself with the skill and then keep the instructions nearby in case you wish to refer to them as you practice. Alternatively, read aloud and record the instructions and listen to it.

Instructions

1. Pick a small object that can rest on a table, is safe to touch, and is emotionally neutral, not charged, such as something your ex gave you. It can be anything: a clock, a pen, a cup. Find a comfortable, quiet place to sit where you won't be disturbed for a few minutes. Place the small object in front of you.

2. Take several slow, deep breaths. Then, without touching the object, look at it and slowly explore its different surfaces with your eyes. Explore the object with curiosity and interest. Look at the different qualities of the object before you:

   - Is the surface of the object dull or shiny?

   - Is it soft or hard?

   - Is it multicolored or just a single color?

   - What's unique or special about the way it looks?

3. Now, pick up the object and hold it in your hand or reach out and touch the object. Notice the different ways the object feels in your hands or to your touch:

   - Is it smooth or rough?

   - Is it soft or hard?

   - Does it bend or is it rigid?

   - Is the surface flat or uneven?

   - Does it feel different in some areas than in other areas?

   - Is it cool, cold, warm, or hot to the touch?

   - Is it heavy or light in weight?

   - What else do you notice about the way it feels?

4. Continue to explore the object with your eyes and your touch. Breathe slowly and comfortably and don't rush. When your attention wanders from the object and your experience of the object, gently return your attention to it.

Skill: Act Mindfully

This informal mindfulness skill applies a mindful attitude to the big and small things you do every day. Acting mindfully means doing all the things that you normally do in your life, such as taking a shower, climbing the stairs, eating lunch, or hugging someone you love, but doing them while also observing your thoughts, feelings, physical sensations, and actions in the present moment.

The best mindful activities are physical activities—not mental—so that you can observe every detail of the experience. It doesn't matter what activity you choose as long as it's brief, you can do it every day, and you can use all your senses (sight, smell, sound, taste, touch). For example, as you walk from the front door to the kitchen, notice the smells of the house. Observe the pattern in the carpet. Notice the sound you make walking. Notice where you place your keys and the sounds they make as you drop them there.

You might want to use signals to remind you to act mindfully. If you plan to eat breakfast mindfully, make a paper place mat on which you've written "Mindful." If you wish to practice walking mindfully home, pick a house or storefront along the way to remind you to shift to walking mindfully.

You might want to begin with just a single daily activity and practice it for a week, but try to plan activities throughout the day—morning, afternoon, evening—so that you're practicing mindful activities all day long. Later, add another activity and another. Use the Mindful Activities Log to track your activities and your experiences doing them mindfully.

Instructions

1. As you apply mindfulness to these activities, notice any thoughts that enter your mind and then gently return your attention to the sensory details of what you're doing at that moment.

2. Describe your experience and rate on a scale of 0 to 10 (where 10 is extreme enjoyment) your level of enjoyment during the activity.

Mindful Activities Log

Activity	Sunday	Monday	Tuesday	Wednesday	Thursday	Friday	Saturday
Walk dog	Calm, happy (6)			Many birds (5)			Beautiful day (7)

Wrap Up

Mindfulness skills build your capacity to move into the present moment and observe rather than react to your internal experiences. It takes regular and consistent practice over time to build your capacity to shift to a mindful attitude when you wish and with little effort. Application of this mindful attitude to life in the moment can help you decrease stress as well as increase the pleasantness of small daily activities that you take for granted.

In this next chapter, you'll learn simple yet powerful skills to think about your thinking. These thinking skills can be life-altering for some people because once you've learned to think about your thinking, you've learned to improve your life.

CHAPTER 4

Thinking Skills

Have you ever wondered why one person gets very angry when cut off in traffic whereas another person feels mildly frustrated? Or why one person is terrified when giving a presentation to coworkers whereas another person is cool and calm? Well, it usually comes down to the different ways the two people think about the situation. Believe it or not, you have a great deal of control over how you think.

Thinking skills are a set of cognitive strategies that help you identify, evaluate, and respond to the way you think about the events and people in your life. For example, you'll learn to put a thought on trial, a skill that you can apply to most thoughts regardless of the emotion or problem. Similarly, you'll learn to identify thinking errors and test thoughts with experiments.

These skills are *inside skills* because they target the thoughts that influence your feelings and actions.

Why Are Thinking Skills Important?

Cognitive behavior therapy assumes that intense negative emotions, such as anxiety, depression, and anger, are maintained through unhelpful and often illogical thinking processes (Beck 1970; 1976; Beck, Emery, and Greenberg 1985; Beck, Rush, Shaw, and Emery 1979). Learning skills to evaluate and respond to unhelpful thinking helps in two ways:

- **Thinking skills dim intense feelings:** Feelings or emotions are completely normal and helpful. Even intense emotions on occasion are normal and helpful as long as they're not so intense and so enduring that they make your life more difficult. If you've ever experienced a panic attack, you know what an intense feeling is like.

Similarly, if you struggle with depression, you experience intense feelings of sadness that persist over time. Learning skills to think differently can decrease the intensity and duration of negative feelings so that you feel better in the moment and throughout the day.

- **Thinking skills increase willingness:** As you learn to dampen intense feelings by thinking about your thinking, you may be more willing to change your actions too. Most people with intense and persistent negative feelings tend to avoid these feelings and the situations that trigger them. It's avoiding feelings rather than the feelings themselves that disrupts life. For example, if you feel intensely and persistently anxious because you worry excessively about what people think of you, then you might avoid the anxiety by declining to attend social events or give important presentations. Avoiding your anxiety in these situations can disrupt your personal and professional lives. Thinking skills that dampen the intensity of negative feelings will increase your willingness to face uncomfortable feelings, and thereby engage in life and prosper.

How to Think About Your Thinking

The process of thinking about your thinking involves three steps:

1. **Identify:** Learning to think about your thinking depends on your ability to identify the particular negative thoughts and unhelpful thought patterns that maintain the negative emotions that create problems in your life.

2. **Evaluate:** Learning to think about your thinking involves evaluating the helpfulness and reasonableness of a thought or thought pattern. Problematic feelings and actions rest on habitual and inflexible patterns of negative thinking.

3. **Respond:** The process of thinking about your thinking concludes with responding to the negative automatic thought with a reasonable, helpful, and accurate view of the situation. Typically, this is an alternative statement that you use to repeatedly respond to problematic automatic thoughts as they arise in the moment. By repeatedly responding to negative automatic thoughts with reasonable (coping) statements, you dim or interrupt the escalation of negative feelings.

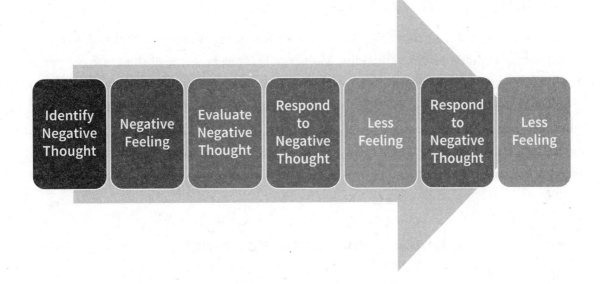

Process of applying thinking skills

Automatic Thoughts

Automatic thoughts are part of our stream of thinking (Beck 1964). They influence our feelings and actions. Our minds generate automatic thoughts all the time, even when we sleep, but most of the time we have little awareness of them, particularly when our attention is engaged elsewhere. Automatic thoughts can be positive (such as "Wow, I had a great time"), neutral, or negative (such as "I can't do anything right").

Thinking skills focus on negative automatic thoughts because they're the thoughts that create the negative feelings you wish to challenge and change. However, people who are persistently in distress are not always aware of the role their negative thinking plays in how they feel and act. Learning to identify, evaluate, and respond to negative automatic thoughts is a great place to focus your thinking skills because changing these thoughts can dramatically improve your mood and functioning.

Identify Automatic Thoughts

You can learn the best thinking skills in the world, but they're useless if you don't know the thoughts on which to focus the skills. Most people are very aware of the physical experience of a feeling, such as a racing heart when you're feeling anxious, or fatigued, and slowed when you're feeling depressed. However, many people are completely unaware of what they're thinking when they're feeling negative feelings, such as anxiety, depression, anger, or guilt. With a bit of practice, you can improve your awareness of these thoughts and their relationships to how you feel and act.

Unpack Emotional Experiences

According to the cognitive behavioral model that you learned in the introduction of this workbook, your automatic thoughts or interpretations of situations create negative feelings (including physical reactions), followed by problematic actions or behaviors. For this reason, different people will have different interpretations of the same situation, and then feel and act differently:

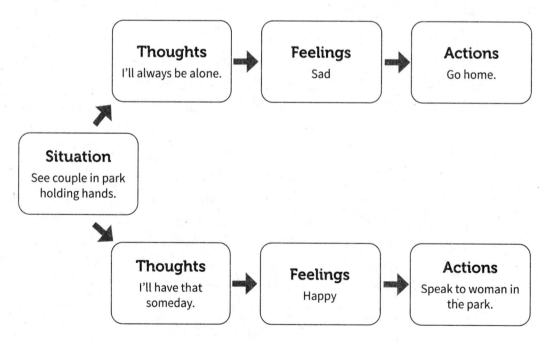

The cognitive behavioral model example

One of the easiest ways to improve your ability to identify negative automatic thoughts is to unpack several recent episodes or events that triggered negative feelings or problematic actions, such as procrastination or unassertiveness. Use the Unpack Emotional Experiences Worksheet to practice this exercise.

Instructions

1. Close your eyes and imagine a recent situation in which you were feeling anxious, angry, sad, or any negative feeling. Try to recall the details of the situation (what was happening, who was there, the time of day). Identifying the specifics of the situation can help you recall the specific automatic thoughts. Describe the situation.

2. Now, follow the feeling. Ask yourself what you were feeling in that situation. Feelings are generally one word, such as "anxious," "angry," or "sad." Thoughts, on the other hand, are usually several words, such as "What if I'm late," "He did it on purpose," or "I can't do anything right." Ask yourself what was going through your mind at that time. Try to identify the thoughts (and images) that arose between the situation and the feeling. Describe the thoughts or images.

3. Describe the feeling. Don't forget to describe your physical reactions, if any. Were you trembling? Were you foggy-headed? Were you clinching your teeth? Also, rate the strength of the feeling from 1 to 10, where 10 is extreme. Write this number next to the feeling.

4. Now, what did you do? Remember, actions follow feelings. Did you walk away? Did you say yes when you wanted to say no? Did you put off starting something? Describe what you did (or didn't do).

5. Repeat this exercise by recalling a situation in which you had a positive feeling, such as happiness, excitement, or contentment.

6. Now, try it with several recent events. You may want to check your goals to identify relevant events. For example, if your goal is to feel less anxious when speaking with people you don't know well, think back to a time recently when that happened.

Unpack Emotional Experiences Worksheet			
Situation	Thoughts	Feelings and Physical Reactions	Actions
Left the end-of-month sales summary on desk of my boss at end of day yesterday.	When he sees that our sales numbers are down this month, he'll fire me for sure.	Anxious, sweating, tense, and fidgeting.	I avoid my boss all day.

Skill: Record Emotional Experiences

Recording the parts (thoughts, feelings, and actions) of your emotional experiences over time increases your awareness of these internal experiences in the same way that writing down your dreams on awakening helps you recall your dreams over time. Through recording, you build your capacity to quickly identify the negative automatic thoughts that fuel your negative emotions. This is critical if you're to benefit from the next steps in the process of learning to think about your thinking: evaluate and respond. Use the Emotional Experiences Log to keep track of these episodes.

Instructions

1. Describe a situation or an event that brought on negative automatic thoughts.

2. Describe your thoughts, feelings, and actions that happened during that situation.

Emotional Experiences Log			
Situation	Thoughts	Feelings	Actions
John is reading the newspaper at breakfast.	He's ignoring me.	Angry (5)	Call him selfish and leave in a huff.

Describe what it was like to identify automatic thoughts and images. Describe anything that surprised you.

_____

_____

_____

_____

Evaluate Automatic Thoughts

Now that you can identify a negative automatic thought, it's time to learn to evaluate whether a thought is true or helpful. There are many skills to evaluate negative automatic thoughts. You'll learn several that work with most negative automatic thoughts.

Skill: Evaluate Costs vs. Benefits of an Automatic Thought

There are costs and benefits to believing a thought is true, and it's important that you understand the costs of continuing to believe something that isn't true but "feels" true in the moment. Look at the example worksheet and then choose a negative automatic thought of your own to evaluate with the Evaluate Costs vs. Benefits of a Thought Worksheet.

Instructions

1. Check your Emotional Experiences Log for a negative automatic thought or think back to a recent situation in which you were feeling a negative emotion.

2. List the costs and benefits of believing the automatic thought is true. To do this, ask yourself:

   - What would change if I believed this thought less?

   - What would change if I believed this thought more?

   - What would change if I believed an alternative to this thought that was more helpful or reasonable?

3. Next to each cost and benefit, assign an importance value, from 1 to 10 (1 = not at all important and 10 = extremely important).

4. Now develop an alternative automatic thought that is more reasonable or helpful. Then list the costs and benefits of believing the alternative thought is true. Then assign importance values to these costs and benefits.

Evaluate Costs vs. Benefits of a Thought Worksheet

Describe negative automatic thought to evaluate: If I ask Daisy out she'll reject me.

Costs	Importance		Benefits	Importance
I'll never get a date with Daisy.	10		I won't be surprised if she rejects me.	3
I settle for someone I like less	8		I avoid rejection.	6
My self-esteem continues to be low.	7			
Total:	25		*Total:*	9

Describe alternative automatic thought to evaluate: Although I can't know ahead of time whether Daisy will reject me, there's no way I'll get a date with her if I don't ask her out.

Costs	Importance		Benefits	Importance
I feel anxious on the first date.	8		Daisy might say yes.	10
			I get more comfortable asking girls out.	8
			Big self-esteem boost if she says yes.	8
			Even if she says no, I might still make a friend.	8
Total:	8		*Total:*	34

Evaluate Costs vs. Benefits of a Thought Worksheet

Describe negative automatic thought to evaluate:

Costs	Importance	Benefits	Importance
Total:		Total:	

Describe alternative automatic thought to evaluate:

Costs	Importance	Benefits	Importance
Total:		Total:	

If at the end of this process you decided that the negative automatic thought works for you, this means that you're willing to absorb the costs of continuing to believe that this thought is true. It's your choice. You can continue to believe any thought you want as long as you're prepared to accept the costs of believing it.

If you've decided that absorbing the costs of continuing to believe the thought works for you, describe why.

_____

_____

_____

_____

_____

_____

_____

Skill: Identify Thinking Errors

People who experience persistent emotional distress tend to make the same errors in thinking over and over. Identifying thinking errors is a quick way to evaluate the reasonableness of an automatic thought. After all, once you understand that a thought is a thinking error, why would you continue to act as if the thought were true? Identifying a thought as a thinking error can quickly create a bit of psychological distance from your thought, which can then dampen what you feel in the moment. Here are several common thinking errors.

Thinking Errors	
1.	*Blaming:* You tend to blame yourself or others for how you feel and without considering your responsibility for changing your feelings or your actions. Or you take complete responsibility for the actions and attitudes of others without considering their role. For example: "My mother caused all my problems." "It's my fault that my son is unhappy."
2.	*Catastrophizing:* You tend to believe that what's happened or will happen will be so horrible that you won't be able to handle it. For example: "I can't handle my anxiety." "It would be horrible if I fail this exam."
3.	*Dichotomous thinking:* You tend to view a person, a situation, or an event in all-or-nothing terms, forcing them to fit only two extreme categories instead of on a continuum. For example: "Everyone hates me." "School is a total waste of time." "I made a mistake, therefore I'm a failure." "I blew my diet completely because I ate more than I planned."
4.	*Discounting the positive:* You tend to discount or minimize your accomplishments or positive attributes or those of others. For example: "I did well because the test was easy." "People like me because they're nice, not because I'm that special." "Attending college isn't a big deal, anyone can do it."
5.	*Emotional reasoning:* You tend to believe that your emotions reflect reality and let them guide your attitudes and judgments. For example: "I feel depressed because my relationship isn't working." "I feel like she doesn't love me, so it must be true." "I'm terrified of flying on airplanes, so flying must be dangerous."
6.	*Fortune telling:* You tend to predict the future but in negative terms and believe that what happens will be so horrible that you won't be able to handle it. For example: "Things will never improve for me." "I'll fail the test and that will be horrible." "I'll be so upset with myself that I won't be able to concentrate for the exam."
7.	*Jumping to conclusions:* You tend to draw conclusions (negative or positive) from little or no confirming evidence. For example: "As soon as I saw him I knew he was going to blame me for being late." "She was looking at me, so I knew she thought it was my fault."
8.	*Labeling:* You tend to assign fixed, global negative labels to yourself and others. For example: "I'm an idiot." "I'm worthless." "She's a terrible friend." "My boss is a horrible manager." "She's a complete jerk."

9.	*Mind reading:* You believe that you know the thoughts and intentions of others (or that they know your thoughts and intentions) without sufficient evidence. Furthermore, you tend to assume that their thoughts or intentions are negative. For example: "He thinks I'm boring." "She knows I'm busy. Why does she keep talking to me?"
10.	*Negative filter:* You tend to focus on the negatives and seldom notice the positives about yourself, others, or events. For example: "No one at this party likes me." "People are rude." "This meeting is pointless."
11.	*Overgeneralization:* You tend to conclude something bigger about yourself or about a single incident with words such as "always," "never," "every," or "only." For example: "I *always* miss the bus." "I failed the math quiz. I can *never* do math." "*Every* time I have a day off from work, it rains." "She *only* says hello when she wants something from me."
12.	*Personalization:* You tend to assume that the actions of others or external events concern (or are directed toward) you without considering other explanations. For example: "It's all my fault that we lost the game" (without considering that other team members made mistakes). "The cashier doesn't like me because she didn't smile at me" (without considering that the cashier didn't smile at anyone).
13.	*Regret bias:* You tend to focus on what you could have done better in the past rather than what you could do better now. For example: "I could have been a better husband." "I shouldn't have said that at the party."
14.	*Shoulds:* You tend to tell yourself that events, the actions of others, and your attitude should (or must, need to, ought to, or have to) be the way you expected or wished them to be rather than how they really are. For example: "I should have given a better presentation." "I have to get an A on this exam." "I should have been a better father."
15.	*Tunnel vision:* You tend to focus on one or a few details and fail to see the whole picture. You're either smart or stupid. Others are either superior or inferior. Events are either good or bad. For example: "The group said that they liked my presentation but since they suggested I add a slide, I know that they didn't really mean it."
16.	*Magnification or minimization:* You tend to magnify the negatives and minimize the positives about yourself, others, and situations. For example: "I got a B on my math test. This shows that I can't do math." "I got an A on my history test. This doesn't mean that I'm smart."

As you read through the list, you may notice that some thinking errors overlap. In fact, some automatic thoughts can contain more than one thinking error. Identifying the particular thinking error for a thought is less important than the fact that you've identified it as a thinking error. A thinking error is an error in thinking, and that's the most important realization. As you practice identifying thinking errors, you'll start to notice that your mind tends to fall into the same pattern of erroneous thinking. Recognizing your erroneous thinking patterns can help you quickly step out of the negative feeling to see things as they really are. Use the Identify Thinking Errors Worksheet to practice this skill.

Instructions

1. Check your Emotional Experiences Log for a negative automatic thought or think back to a recent situation in which you were feeling a negative emotion.

2. Read the list of thinking errors. Next to the automatic thought, write the number of the thinking error that fits the automatic thought.

3. As you continue to record your automatic thoughts in the Emotional Experiences Log, write the thinking error numbers next to each automatic thought.

Identify Thinking Errors Worksheet		
Situation	**Automatic Thoughts**	**Thinking Errors**
My boss didn't comment on my presentation.	He thought it was terrible. He's going to fire me for sure.	9, 7, 2

Describe the particular types of thinking errors you tend to make.

_____

_____

_____

Skill: Put an Automatic Thought on Trial

This thinking skill is a fun and effective way to evaluate a negative automatic thought. You'll put a thought on trial as you act as defense attorney, prosecuting attorney, and judge. As the defense and prosecuting attorneys, you'll gather evidence in support of or against the negative automatic thought. Evidence is a verifiable fact. Evidence is not an interpretation, opinion, or guess. As the judge, you'll come to a verdict regarding the negative automatic thought. Is the thought accurate or reasonable? The verdict is the alternative response to the situation.

The goal of this skill is to decrease how strongly you believe a thought through precise evaluation of objective evidence. Think through the evidence carefully. It's more effective to ask yourself questions than it is to tell yourself what is or isn't reasonable (Braun, Strunk, Sasso, and Cooper 2015; Heiniger, Clark, and Egan 2018). In other words, your goal is to place a question mark behind a thought. You'll know the question mark is there when you think to yourself, "Gee, I've never thought about it that way before." Look at the example worksheet and then choose a negative thought of your own to evaluate with the Put a Thought on Trial Worksheet.

Instructions

1. Write the negative automatic thought you'll put on trial under *Thought on Trial*.

2. Rate how strongly you believe the thought to be true and the strength of your feeling (e.g., anxiety, anger, or sadness).

3. Check the list of thinking errors from the previous skill. Identify all the thinking errors for the thought on trial. Enter these under *Thinking Errors*.

4. In *The Defense* column, describe all the objective evidence that the thought is true (or mostly true). Evidence is a verifiable fact. It's not an opinion, assumption, or guess. Ask yourself these questions regarding the thought about the situation:

   - Could there be any other explanations?

   - What's the evidence that this thought is true?

   - Is the situation really so important?

   - What would I tell a friend who was in this situation?

- Is there a more helpful way to think about this?

- Is there another explanation that better fits the evidence?

- Am I 100 percent certain this event or consequence will happen? Why not?

- Have I looked at this same situation in a different way in the past? Did that help?

- Is this explanation true for everyone in my situation?

5. In *The Prosecution* column, describe all the objective evidence the thought is false (or mostly false).

6. As the judge, step back and consider the evidence. Summarize the evidence and enter this in *The Judge's Verdict*.

7. Re-rate how strongly you believe the thought to be true and the strength of your feeling.

8. If the thought that's on trial is a prediction, consider creating an experiment to test whether the prediction is true or false. You'll learn to do this in the Test Automatic Thoughts with Experiments skill that follows.

Put a Thought on Trial Worksheet

Thought on Trial I'm a horrible salesperson.

Strength of Belief (0–100%):	90%	Strength of Feeling (0–10):	7

Thinking Errors #10 Negative filter, #4 Discounting the positive, #3 Dichotomous thinking

The Defense	The Prosecution
My boss told me that he was disappointed that we didn't get the sale. I missed my monthly sales target a couple of months ago.	Last month, my boss gave me a raise and I got the Rising Star award. I've made my annual sales target three years running. The other salespeople are having an off month. My performance evaluations have always been excellent!

The Judge's Verdict

Although my sales are down, my boss tells me that I'm an excellent salesperson. It's not realistic to expect to perform always at 100%. I don't control the economy or what products we're told to push. I'm not perfect, but I'm still a good salesperson!

Strength of Belief (0–100%):	60%	Strength of Feeling (0–10):	4

Put a Thought on Trial Worksheet

Thought on Trial

Strength of Belief (0–100%):		Strength of Feeling (0–10):	

Thinking Errors

The Defense	**The Prosecution**

The Judge's Verdict

Strength of Belief (0–100%):		Strength of Feeling (0–10):	

Skill: Test Automatic Thoughts with Experiments

Even after evaluating an automatic thought you may still believe it to be true to some degree, particularly when you're experiencing intense feelings in the moment. That's because evaluating an automatic thought only places a question mark behind the thought. Behavioral experiments (Bennett-Levy 2003; Bennett-Levy et al. 2004) are a powerful way to evaluate thoughts on a deep level because you test your thoughts in the real world, as opposed to hypothetically testing them, as you do with the Put a Thought on Trial skill.

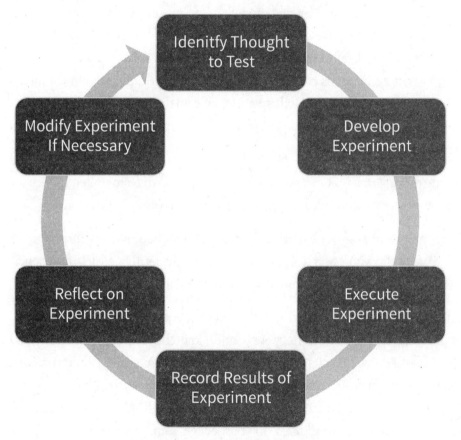

Process of testing a thought

The process of testing a thought involves identifying a thought to test; devising and planning an experiment to test it; executing the experiment; and then reflecting on and learning from the experiment. Look at the example worksheet and then choose a negative thought of your own to evaluate with the Test a Thought Worksheet.

Instructions

1. Identify an unreasonable or helpful *thought to test*. Typically, testable thoughts are predictions or expectations about events. Ask yourself, "What is my prediction?" "What do I expect will happen?

2. *Rate* how strongly (0 to 100 percent, where 100 percent is completely) you believe the thought is true (the prediction will happen).

3. Design an *experiment* to test the thought. The most effective experiments are those that you can tell objectively whether the prediction was confirmed or not confirmed. Identify how you'll tell *whether the prediction is true*. Ask yourself, "How will I know whether the prediction is true?" For example, rather than "No one will like me at the party," try instead "No one will speak to me at the party." If evidence that no one likes you at the party is that no one speaks to you at the party, then you've developed a testable prediction.

4. *Execute the experiment*. Observe what really happened. Remember, evidence is not an opinion of what you think happened but what you observed happen.

5. *Review* the results of the experiment. What happened? Was your prediction true or false? What did you observe that confirmed or disconfirmed it? If a friend observed the experiment, would they have observed the same thing?

6. *Reflect* on what you learned from the experiment. Focus on what you expected to happen versus what really happened and how the original thought changed as a result. Based on the results of the experiment, is there a new or alternative view that might be more accurate and helpful? How could you test the alternative view or prediction? If you repeated the experiment, how strongly (0 to 100 percent, where 100 percent is completely confident) do you believe your prediction will happen then? If the strength changed, why? Would you change the experiment in any way to clarify the results or answer another question? What do you want to remember? What did you learn that surprised you?

7. *Re-rate* how strongly (0 to 100 percent, where 100 percent is completely) you believe the thought is true.

Test a Thought Worksheet	
Thought to Test	If I don't take a nap every day then I can't function.
Rate	90%
Experiment	I won't nap at all for one week, starting today.
How I Will Know the Thought Is True	I won't be able to do my job: answer the phones, stay awake in meetings, direct calls to the right people. On a 0–100 scale, I will function about a 50.
Review	I answered phones and replied appropriately, I stayed awake in all the meetings, I directed the calls to the right people, and I caught several mistakes that my coworker made. On the 0–100 scale, I functioned about a 75. I was tired but I did okay.
Reflect	I guess it means that I can function okay even if I don't nap. In fact, this last week with no naps I slept a little better.
Re-rate	40%

Test a Thought Worksheet	
Thought to Test	
Rate	
Experiment	
How I Will Know the Thought Is True	
Review	
Reflect	
Re-rate	

Describe what it was like to think about thoughts as predictions or expectations to test with experiments.

_____

_____

_____

_____

_____

_____

_____

_____

_____

At times, you may wish to test predictions about feelings (anxious, sad, angry, guilty, pleasant). Describe your prediction about the feeling. How intensely (0–10) do you predict you'll feel? How many times do you predict it will go that high per day (per hour, per week)? How long do you predict you'll feel this level of distress? One minute, thirty minutes, an hour, all day? For example, "The intensity of my embarrassment will be 10 out of 10 and stay at that level for the entire week."

Skill: Look Through the Lens of Time

Emotional reasoning is a thinking error that tends to amplify feelings. That's because when something upsets you, you tend to look at the event through an emotional lens that makes it feel like the most important event in the world. But transporting yourself into the future and looking back at the event through the lens of time can help you feel better. Whatever seemed end-of-the-world important when it happened can feel less important after some time has passed. Look at the example worksheet and then choose an event of your own to evaluate with the Look Through the Lens of Time Worksheet.

Instructions

1. Describe the event that upset you.

2. Rate how important the event feels now. Use an importance scale of 0 to 10 (0 = it's not at all important, 5 = it's important but not life-changing, and 10 = your life depends on it).

3. Rate how important the event will feel in an hour and then a day (week, month, year, five years, and ten years).

4. Re-rate how important the event feels after you completed the exercise.

5. Reflect on the event. Write this new view under *How You Think About the Event Now*.

Look Through the Lens of Time Worksheet

Event That Upset You: My girlfriend broke up with me.	
Rate how important (0–10) this event feels at the moment:	9
Ask yourself the following questions and re-rate the importance (0–10) each time:	
How important will this event feel in an hour?	9
How important will this event feel in a day?	7
How important will this event feel in a week?	5
How important will this event fell in a month?	3
How important will this event feel in a year?	1
How important will this event feel in five years?	0
How important will this event feel in ten years?	0
Re-rate how important this event feels now:	3
How You Think About the Event Now: Well, the breakup hurt deeply in the moment, but I'll heal. It just takes some time and each week I'll feel a little better. I know that's true.	

Look Through the Lens of Time Worksheet

Event That Upset You:	
Rate how important (0–10) this event feels at the moment:	
Ask yourself the following questions and re-rate the importance (0–10) each time:	
How important will this event feel in an hour?	
How important will this event feel in a day?	
How important will this event feel in a week?	
How important will this event fell in a month?	
How important will this event feel in a year?	
How important will this event feel in five years?	
How important will this event feel in ten years?	
Re-rate how important this event feels now:	
How You Think About the Event Now:	

Respond to Automatic Thoughts

The final step in thinking about your thinking is to respond to negative automatic thoughts with rational or reasonable statements or summaries of the facts. For example, rational statements from evaluating negative automatic thoughts in the previous skills might include:

- Statement of the costs of believing an automatic thought is true. For example, "Although I can't know ahead of time whether Daisy will reject me, there's no way I'll get a date with her if I don't ask her out."

- Statement that a thought is a thinking error. For example, "I'm mind reading now. I really don't know what she's thinking. Why jump to the conclusion that she's upset with me when I don't know that it's true or not?"

- Statement that summarizes the evidence that a thought is not true (Judge's verdict). For example, "Although my sales are down, my boss tells me that I'm an excellent salesperson. It's not realistic to expect to perform always at 100 percent. I don't control the economy or what products we're told to push. I'm not perfect, but I'm still a good salesperson!"

- Statement that summarizes what you learned in an experiment you completed to test whether a thought was true or not. For example, "I guess it means that I can function okay even if I don't nap. In fact, this last week with no naps, I slept a little better."

- Statement that summarizes what you learned from looking through the lens of time. For example, "Well, the breakup hurt deeply in the moment, but I'll heal. It just takes some time and each week I'll feel a little better. I know that's true."

Write your rational responses or statements on an index card or enter them in your phone. The goal is to repeatedly respond to the negative automatic thought when it arises in the moment or read through the rational statements before you enter a situation. For example, you might read through your rational statement prior to giving a presentation to help you feel less anxious or when you think about your recent breakup to feel less down.

Another option is to rehearse applying the coping or rational statement in your mind before you use it in the real world. You'll learn to do this in chapter 9. It's a great way to build your confidence that the rational statement works, and it increases the likelihood that you'll use it when it counts: in real life.

Describe several rational responses you developed with the skills you've learned and the situations in which you'll use them:

_____

_____

_____

_____

_____

_____

_____

Wrap Up

Perhaps there is no more important CBT skill than learning to think about your thinking. That's because you have a great deal more control over how you think than over how you feel. Learning to identify, evaluate, and respond to unhelpful negative automatic thoughts can dim intense feelings and increase your willingness to change your behavior, which is the foundation of deep learning and change.

In the next chapter, you'll learn skills to improve and protect your relationships with others. Caring and supportive relationships are essential to our well-being, yet they require nurturing. These interpersonal effectiveness skills are easy to learn and, when practiced regularly, can build resilient relationships that insulate you from the hard knocks of life.

CHAPTER 5

Interpersonal Effectiveness Skills

Caring and supportive relationships are essential to our well-being. Through our relationships, we learn to love and be loved. They're a source of companionship and inspiration. They help us navigate difficult times and make life worth living. Yet through carelessness or indifference, we can damage our relationships, sometimes beyond repair. In this chapter, you'll learn skills to improve and protect your relationships with others. Whether it's standing up for yourself or communicating clearly, interpersonal effectiveness skills can improve the quality of your personal and professional relationships.

Interpersonal effectiveness skills (Linehan 2014) are a set of social strategies to help you manage interpersonal interactions that contribute to difficulties with others. In the previous chapter, you learned thinking skills that target problems with perception. Interpersonal effectiveness skills target problems in the social world around you and are therefore *outside skills*.

Why Are Interpersonal Skills Important?

Interpersonal effectiveness skills are important for several reasons. First, they build and sustain strong relationships with others, which makes life more enjoyable and meaningful. Second, interpersonal effectiveness skills dampen your emotional responses to interpersonal events. For example, communication skills can increase your social confidence, and with greater social confidence, you'll feel less anxious and distressed in your relationships with others. There are many interpersonal effectiveness skills and the ones presented here primarily focus on listening and responding, resolving conflict, and assertiveness.

At the same time, as helpful as these interpersonal skills are, their effectiveness also depends on your ability to regulate your emotions (anxiety, anger, sadness, guilt). You've learned many of those skills in the previous chapters and you can use those skills while you work on the skills in this chapter. For example, you might apply the 4-7-8 breathing that you learned to calm your emotional system as you practice assertiveness if speaking up makes you anxious.

Identify Your Interpersonal Strengths and Weaknesses

Not everyone interacts well with every person all the time in every circumstance. We all have our strengths and weaknesses when it comes to interacting with others. Knowing what you do well and not so well will help you focus on the interpersonal effectiveness skills that can help you the most. Take a moment to consider your interpersonal skills with the Identify Your Interpersonal Strengths and Weaknesses Worksheet.

Instructions

1. Place a check (✔) next to the statements that best reflect how you act and react in typical interpersonal situations.

2. Add the even-numbered statements and add the odd-numbered statements. If the total of even-numbered statements is higher, then your interpersonal skills are adequate in typical situations with others. If the total of odd-numbered statements is higher, then you can benefit from learning and applying a few more interpersonal skills with others.

		Identify Your Interpersonal Strengths and Weaknesses
	1.	I assume people know what I'm trying to say.
	2.	After the other person speaks, I clarify what I heard them say before I respond.
	3.	When speaking with someone, I tend to finish sentences for the other person.
	4.	I let the other person finish speaking before I react to what they say.
	5.	It's difficult for me to accept constructive criticism for another person.
	6.	When someone hurts my feelings, I discuss this with them.
	7.	It's difficult for me to admit to someone that I'm wrong or I've made a mistake.
	8.	I apologize easily to someone if I've hurt their feelings.
	9.	People tend to become defensive when I disagree with them or share my opinion.
	10.	I tend to show interest by smiling and leaning forward when speaking with people.
	11.	It's difficult for me to talk to people I don't know well.
	12.	It's easy for me to stand up for myself if someone is taking advantage of me.
	13.	People tend to misunderstand what I'm saying or where I'm coming from.
	14.	I'm good at summarizing the key points of conversations I have with other people.
	15.	I tend to get in someone's face when I'm upset by something they said to me.
	16.	I don't plan my response or comeback while the other person is speaking.
	17.	I have trouble asking people for simple things, such as asking for directions.
	18.	I'm open-minded and I'm willing to change my opinion based on others' views.
	19.	I tend to avoid conflict with other people if I can.
	20.	I tend to nod and smile to signal that I'm listening and encourage others to speak.
	21.	People tell me that I'm shouting at them when I'm just trying to tell them how I feel.
	22.	I can keep cool when speaking to people even when they're upset with me.
	23.	When I disagree with someone about something, the situation often escalates.
	24.	I'm good at getting my point across to other people.
	25.	I tend to go along with other people's requests rather than negotiating with them.
	26.	I don't shout or point at people during heated conversations.

Total Even-Numbered Statements	Total Odd-Numbered Statements

Describe the typical interpersonal situations (for example, saying no to your sister when she makes an unreasonable request, resolving conflicts or disagreements with your coworkers, asking your friends for favors) you handle well and those you'd like to handle better and why.

_____

_____

_____

_____

_____

_____

_____

_____

Communication Skills

There is a clear and positive relationship between effective interpersonal communication skills and a range of benefits, such as greater happiness in life, resilience to stress and psychosocial problems, and enhanced academic and professional achievements (Hannawa and Spitzberg 2015; Müller et al. 2015; Hargie 2017).

Communication skills include a range of strategies to build and maintain social relationships. This chapter presents those that are the most important in supporting your social well-being as well as the social well-being of others.

Skill: Listen and Respond

How many times has someone said to you, "You're not hearing me." Well, you likely heard them but didn't respond in a way that communicated that you did. In fact, you may have heard them and disagreed with them but you didn't communicate that either. The point is that effective communication is an active process. It isn't just about listening. It's about responding in a way that signals that you heard what the person said. This is called active listening. To listen actively, follow these three steps:

Instructions

1. **Listen carefully to what the person said to you.** Listening carefully is an important skill in all your interactions, but when the interaction is heated, it's essential. Intense emotions make listening, not hearing, difficult because it takes effort to pay attention to what the other person is saying when you feel anxious or angry or guilty or sad. You're caught up in the emotion as you try to think of a comeback or counterargument. At the same time, you're working hard to remain calm. That takes attention too, and it's necessary that you remain calm in order to listen to what the other person is really saying. When you listen actively, it not only helps you pay attention to what the other person is saying, but you'll also actually take in what they're saying.

2. **Repeat back what the person said to you.** To avoid misunderstandings, it helps to repeat back what the person said to you. You can repeat back what the person said in two ways. You can repeat exactly what the person said or you can paraphrase what the person said. When you paraphrase, you don't repeat back the same words like a parrot. Instead, you repeat an approximation of what the person said.

3. **Clarify the point or problem the person made.** Jumping to the wrong conclusion often results in upset and needless arguments. Clarifying or checking your assumptions about the point or problem helps you check that you have the correct information before you respond. Even if you have different takes or opinions about the topic, you'll understand where the person is coming from.

Like most things, it takes practice to get good at listening and responding. A great way to practice is with a close friend or family member. Just ask them a question and then listen and respond actively.

Skill: Use I-Messages

When you listen to people, you'll hear either You-messages or I-messages, and You-messages make communicating with someone, particularly during a conflict or intense emotions, much more difficult. You-messages put people on the defensive, particularly when you use words such as "should," "must," "ought to," "need to," "always," and "never." When you say to a friend, "You should watch this new show," it might sound as if you're telling them that they're out of touch for not watching it. When you send a You-message, people stop listening and wait for the attack or put-down. Here are a couple of examples:

Situation: Your boyfriend is late picking you up for the movie.

You-Message: You are always late!

Situation: Your boss asked you to work Saturday again.

You-Message: You never consider that I have a life outside of work.

I-messages, on the other hand, help you clearly and honestly express yourself without blaming others. When you send an I-message, you take responsibility for how you think and feel, which is less likely to put someone on the defensive. I-messages put people at ease because it sounds as if it's about you and not about them, even when sometimes it is about them. There are three parts to I-messages:

1. I feel…

2. When you…

3. Because…

Take a look at the examples in the Practice Using I-Messages Worksheet and then add your own.

Instructions

1. Think about a situation in which you want to communicate with I-messages.

2. Write the three parts to your I-message.

Practice Using I-Messages Worksheet

Situation	My sister borrowed my sweater without asking first.
I feel...	Upset
...when you...	Borrow my things without asking my permission
...because...	I think you don't respect me
All together	I feel upset when you borrow my things without asking my permission because I think you don't respect me.
Situation	
I feel...	
...when you...	
...because...	
All together	
Situation	
I feel...	
...when you...	
...because...	
All together	

Identify Your Communication Style

Passive and aggressive communication styles tend to undermine your effectiveness in many interpersonal situations. A passive communication style may work in the short term. It's easier to go along with what the other person wants, or to say yes, regardless of how unreasonable the request may be. In the long term, however, a passive communication style tends to create a life in which you're unfulfilled, unhappy, and resentful. And that resentment can build until you explode and perhaps damage the relationship forever.

At the other end of communication styles is aggressive communication. That's a style in which you yell or threaten or intimidate the other person. As you can imagine, not too many relationships can weather over time aggressive communication. Use the Identify Your Communication Style Worksheet to examine your style.

Instructions

1. Think back to several recent interactions with friends, family members, or coworkers. Place a check (✓) next to the statements that best fit your typical interaction in the situation.

2. Add the even-numbered statements and add the odd-numbered statements. If the total of even-numbered statements is higher, then your typical interpersonal style is *passive*. If the total of odd-numbered statements is higher, then your typical interpersonal style is *assertive*.

		Identify Your Communication Style Worksheet
	1.	When someone treats me unfairly, I call it to their attention.
	2.	I find it difficult to make decisions.
	3.	I'm openly critical of someone's opinions, ideas, or behaviors.
	4.	When someone cuts in front of me in line, I don't mention it to them.
	5.	I insist that my spouse or roommate do their fair share of household chores.
	6.	When a salesperson tries to sell me something, I find it hard to say no.
	7.	I point out to a salesperson when they serve a latecomer before me.
	8.	I'm reluctant to speak up in a discussion or debate.
	9.	I mention to a person who has borrowed money or other possessions if it's overdue.
	10.	It's difficult for me to express what I feel to someone.
	11.	I'm comfortable if someone gives me direct feedback.
	12.	I find it difficult to keep eye contact when talking to another person.
	13.	When my meal is improperly prepared, I ask the sever to correct the situation.
	14.	I'm uncomfortable if someone watches me at work.
	15.	When someone is kicking or bumping my chair, I ask the person to stop.
	16.	When I discover merchandise is faulty, I seldom return it.
	17.	I insist that a repair person make repairs or replacements that are their responsibility.
	18.	I seldom step in and make decisions for others.
	19.	I'm able to ask friends for small favors or help.
	20.	When I differ with a person I respect, I'm uncomfortable sharing my own viewpoint.
	21.	I'm able to refuse unreasonable requests made by friends.
	22.	I'm uncomfortable complimenting or praising others.
	23.	If I'm disturbed by someone smoking near me, I can tell them.
	24.	When I meet a stranger, I'm usually not the first to introduce myself.

Total Even-Numbered Statements	Total Odd-Numbered Statements

Assertiveness

Both passive and aggressive communication styles destroy relationships. But there's another way. That's assertive communication, and it's a powerful interpersonal effectiveness skill. Assertive communication doesn't guarantee you'll get what you want in your relationships, but it certainly increases the odds when compared to the alternatives: passive or aggressive communication. Assertive communication can help you ask for what you want in relationships, say no and set other limits, and share with people your likes and dislikes. Unlike passive and aggressive communication styles, assertive communication builds and strengthens your relationships.

Assertiveness includes a range of behaviors that help you get along in life and take care of yourself in a variety of ways. Perhaps the two most important assertive actions are making everyday requests and standing your ground.

Skill: Make Everyday Requests

If assertiveness doesn't come easily to you, making everyday requests is a great place to start. Making everyday requests of others, such as asking a stranger for directions or asking the host to seat you at a different table in a restaurant, helps you get along in life and enjoy it more too. Similarly, assertive requests, such as asking someone for their opinion about an event or what they like to do for fun, can transform acquaintances into friends. There are four parts to making everyday requests:

1. **Brief explanation (optional):** Many situations don't require any explanation, such as "Please pass the salt." However, when it makes sense to explain why you're making the request, keep it to a single simple sentence.

   "I'm lost…"

   "This box is too heavy for me to carry…"

   "These jeans feel a little tight…"

2. **Softening statement:** This signals to the other person that you're about to make a request and that you're a polite, reasonable person.

"Would you mind…?"

"I was wondering if…"

"I'd appreciate if you would…"

3. **Direct specific question:** You state what you want clearly and specifically. State your request as if it's a normal and reasonable request that anyone would be glad to accommodate. Don't qualify or elaborate. This only makes the request seem unreasonable when it's not.

4. **Appreciative statement:** This encourages the other person to say yes to the request and increases the likelihood that they'll say yes to similar requests in the future. Also, an appreciative statement can make them feel special that they could do this for you.

"This is great of you…"

"I really appreciate…"

"Thanks for doing this…"

When you put the four parts together, your everyday requests can look like these:

"It's a little cold in here. Would you mind turning up the thermostat? Thanks so much."

"I'm a bit confused. I'd appreciate if you'd go over that again. This would really help."

"I'm nervous driving this fast. Would you mind slowing down? Thanks for doing this."

Skill: Stand Your Ground

At times, to feel safe or comfortable, it makes sense to stand your ground, for example, saying no to someone who asks for your number, declining to work another Saturday when your boss insists that you're the only one who can, or telling a friend who is chronically late to arrive on time. There are four parts to the stand your ground skill (DEAL):

1. *Describe the problem.* When you're talking to someone, tell them what the problem is. For example, "This is the third time you've been late to pick me up."

2. *Express how the problem makes you feel without blaming the other person.* For example, "Once or twice is okay, but three times hurts my feelings and makes me think that you don't care."

3. *Ask for a change.* It helps to suggest what the person could do to change or fix the situation. For example, "How about we agree that if you're running late you'll text me so I know what's up."

4. *List how you think the change is going to improve your situation or fix the problem.* This motivates the person to try the proposed solution. For example, "I think that if you let me know when you're running late, then I'll feel less upset because I'll know whether to leave on my own or wait for you."

Now take a few minutes to identify typical everyday situations in which you could practice, for example:

- **With strangers:** When someone cuts in front of you in line. When a server brings you the wrong order. When a cashier gives you the incorrect amount of change.

- **With coworkers or colleagues:** When a coworker borrows your stapler without asking first. When a colleague takes credit for something that you did. When an employee who reports to you misses a work deadline.

- **With friends or family:** When a family member accuses you of something you didn't do. When a friend is late again for a date. When a sibling forgets to return something you loaned them.

- **With teachers or employers:** When your boss asks you to work Saturday again. When a teacher marks a problem on a test wrong when it's correct. When your adviser insists you take a course but you don't think it's necessary to graduate.

Now identify several situations to practice it and write assertiveness scripts for those situations. Scripts help you think through the steps ahead of time so that you're confident and less anxious when the time comes to use them. Also, developing scripts for the typical situations that arise in your life helps you respond assertively with confidence in the moment. Use the DEAL Worksheet to practice this skill.

Instructions

1. Identify at least three situations in which you can practice standing your ground.

   _____

   _____

   _____

   _____

2. Write a script for each one.

DEAL Worksheet	
Situation:	
Describe:	
Express:	
Ask:	
List:	
Situation:	
Describe:	
Express:	
Ask:	
List:	
Situation:	
Describe:	
Express:	
Ask:	
List:	

Skill: Build an Assertiveness Practice Ladder, Then Practice

Assertiveness is a powerful skill, but it's not easy to practice at first. Most unassertive people feel a bit anxious because it can feel risky. That's why it helps to practice in low-risk situations to get your feet wet, build up confidence, and then work toward more anxiety-evoking situations. That's where the Assertiveness Practice Ladder Worksheet comes in.

Instructions

1. Make a list of situations where you want to practice assertiveness. Include problems with friends, family, people who work for you or with you, and so on.

2. Rank the situations from 1 to 10 in terms of risk and difficulty, with 1 being the least challenging and 10 being the most challenging. Try to list situations that cover the ladder in terms of difficulty, with some easier ones and some difficult ones.

3. Write an assertiveness script for each of the situations on the ladder.

4. Practice assertiveness in the first (easiest) situation. After this first practice, reflect on what worked and what you could improve. For example, could you change the script to improve the effectiveness of your assertive statement? Could you stand or act a bit differently to communicate more confidence? Incorporate what you learned and try the second (next easiest) situation.

5. Continue to move up the ladder in this way. It's okay to practice the same situation (same step) several times before you move up to the next step. With each step up the ladder, your confidence builds.

Assertiveness Practice Ladder Worksheet

Rank	Situation
10	
9	
8	
7	
6	
5	
4	
3	
2	
1	

Describe what you observed when you were assertive in these situations and why you think people responded the way they did.

_____

_____

_____

_____

_____

_____

_____

_____

_____

Manage Conflict

It's nearly impossible for two people to agree on everything all the time. Therefore, conflict is inevitable. Managing conflict in healthy ways strengthens and deepens your relationships with friends, family, coworkers, and others. To manage conflict effectively, try these skills:

- Bookend with validation

- Play the broken record

- Agree to disagree

- Pick the flower and ignore the weeds

- Ask for time or a second opinion

Skill: Bookend with Validation

Typically, people move from conversation to conflict when one person doesn't believe they're understood. They then try to get the other person to understand them with more arguments, assertions, and, at times, raised voices. A simple and effective way to de-escalate this cycle is to bookend both sides with validating statements.

Validating someone's point of view doesn't mean you agree with it or them. It means that you understand where they're coming from. A bookend validation begins with an "I understand…" statement that validates the other person's point of view and signals that you get why they think and feel the way they do. This is then followed with an "On my end…" statement that validates your point of view to help the other person understand where you're coming from. Here are some examples:

- "*I understand* that you think there's no way you can finish this project on time. It's a big project with an accelerated schedule. *On my end*, my boss is pressuring me to move this project along as quickly as possible. A lot is riding on this project for both of us."

- "*I understand* that you're trying to keep the house neat and tidy. I appreciate that a lot. *On my end*, it's frustrating when I have to look for something that you put away. It wastes time. A tidy house isn't as important to me as getting things done as quickly as I can."

- "*I understand* that when I said you're not doing your share, it hurt your feelings. It would be hard for me to hear too. *On my end*, I work all day and then come home to see you watching television. I'm not asking you to do everything at home, but I want a little more from you."

Reflect on typical personal and professional situations that arise when you could practice bookending with validation.

_____

_____

_____

_____

_____

_____

_____

_____

_____

_____

Skill: Play the Broken Record

Even when you bookend with validation, people sometimes continue to push back. Rather than continuing to reason with them, which only increases your frustration, try the broken record technique. First, develop a one-sentence, specific, simple statement that states what you want or don't want. Avoid excuses and don't explain yourself. You're past all that. It's broken record time. If the other person asks why (e.g., "Why do you want to…?" "Why is that so important to you?") just say, "That's the way I prefer it" or "That's the way I see it." Answering "why" questions just gives the other person ammunition to continue arguing with you. Send confident body signals: maintain eye contact and speak in a calm and firm voice.

Then just repeat the statement as many times as it takes. Vary a word here or there, but continue the main message. Here's an example:

Jole: I've paid for lunch the last couple of times. I'd like you to pay this time.

Jill: I'm a little short this week. I'll pay next time.

Jole: You and I make about the same salary. I'd like you to pay today.

Jill: Why don't you trust me? Don't you think I'll pay next time?

Jole: I've paid the last few times. It doesn't seem fair. I want you to pay for lunch today.

Jill: Don't get bent out of shape. I said I'd pay next time.

Jole: You haven't paid for lunch in weeks. I'd like you to pay for lunch today.

Skill: Agree to Disagree

This technique signals to the other person that you're finished discussing an issue. Most people—even those who are convinced they're right and that you're wrong—can agree to disagree. For example, "I hear what you're saying. I hope you'll agree to disagree on this one." Or, "We've discussed this for a while now. I think it's time we agree to disagree."

Skill: Pick the Flower and Ignore the Weeds

This strategy is a great way to de-escalate a conflict because you agree in part with what someone is saying. That's the flower. And you ignore the other parts of what someone is saying with which you disagree. That's the weeds. The trick is to find a part—no matter how small—of what they say that you accept. Then communicate to the person that you agree with that part. You ignore the rest of their argument or explanation. Watch for words like "always" and "never." There's likely a small truth in these exaggerations for you to pick:

Other: You always say no when I want to buy something.

You: You're right. I do at times say no when you ask for money.

Other: You never listen to me.

You: It's true. There have been times when I missed something you were saying to me.

Skill: Ask for Time or a Second Opinion

This technique pushes the pause button. It's particularly helpful when someone is pressuring you to make a decision or to agree to a plan right away. Asking for a little time gives you room to cool down and prepare an effective response or counteroffer. For example, "You've made some good points. I always give myself twenty-four hours to think through these kinds of situations. When can I call you tomorrow?" Or, "Let me get back to you after lunch. This is important and I want to think carefully about it before I commit to anything."

Another delay technique is to tell the other person you want a second opinion. Not only does this give you time to think through what you want but it also might help to run the situation by a neutral third party. For example, "I like to bounce this kind of thing off my sales lead before I commit to it. I'll get back to you after I speak with her." Or, "I always run issues like this by my partner before I commit. I'll call you tomorrow after I speak with him."

Skill: Negotiate

Negotiating means that you and another person work to find a compromise or middle ground for a situation or problem. When you and the person reach a compromise, each of you wins a little and loses a little, and that way, you both win. The best negotiations begin before you even meet and speak with the person. Use the Negotiate Worksheet when you are preparing to negotiate a conflict or conflicting needs.

Instructions

1. In the *Give a Little* column, list the things about the situation or problem that you could give a little on.

2. In the *Hold Firm* column, list the things that you want to hold firm on.

3. In the *My Opening Suggestion or Solution* box, write the first solution or suggestion you'll offer as you start to negotiate.

Negotiate Worksheet	
Give a Little	**Hold Firm**
1.	1.
2.	2.
3.	3.
My Opening Suggestion or Solution	

Now that you've prepared to negotiate, it's time to begin the actual negotiation process. If you start the negotiation process, offer the opening suggestion or solution you identified. As the negotiation continues, make sure to offer solutions that address at least some of the concerns of the other person. If you aren't sure what the person wants, then ask, "What do you want from me?" Or, "Where do you think I could give a little?"

During the negotiation, smile and nod your head as you listen to the person. This signals that you're confident there's a middle ground and that you're open to working with the person to find it. During the negotiation, consider one or more of the following compromise strategies:

- **Split the difference:** This works when negotiating about how much time to spend doing something or how much money to spend.

- **Take turns:** This works when negotiating participation in an activity. For example, on a road trip, you drive before lunch and your friend drives after lunch.

- **Trial period:** Agree to a solution for a period of time and then reevaluate. If it's not working for the other person, renegotiate.

- **Exchange this for that:** This is another way to negotiate activities, such as chores. You'll clean the bathroom each week if your roommate vacuums the common areas each week.

- **My way, then your way:** This is a great way for each person to get their way. For example, you get to listen to opera while cooking dinner and your partner gets to listen to heavy metal when cleaning the kitchen after dinner.

Wrap Up

Interpersonal effectiveness skills are vital to building and sustaining strong relationships that make life fun and meaningful. Furthermore, interpersonal effectiveness skills increase confidence that you can take care of yourself in a host of ways.

In the next chapter, you'll learn skills to improve your ability to manage time and tasks. Not only will these skills help you be more effective and productive in life but you'll also feel less stressed as you pursue success.

CHAPTER 6

Time and Task Management Skills

The truth is that we have just twenty-four hours each day. How we spend those hours makes a big difference in how much we get done as well as how rushed and overwhelmed we feel. In this chapter, you'll learn skills to manage time and tasks, and believe it or not, you have more influence over these than you think you do. Whether it's starting homework, replying to emails, completing small assignments and big projects on time, or simply folding laundry, you'll learn skills that will create more peace of mind and extra time to do what is important to you.

Time and task management skills are a set of behavioral strategies that help you start and finish tasks efficiently. These skills are primarily *outside skills* because they target two things that are outside of you: the projects and activities that are part of your life, and the time you have to do them. At the same time, how you think can influence your ability to start tasks, and you'll learn skills to help you with that too.

Why Are Time and Task Management Skills Important?

Even when you're smart and competent, if you lack time and task management skills, two things tend to happen. First, you fall farther and farther behind in life and this can create personal and professional consequences, such as distressed relationships and missed professional opportunities. Second, these real-life consequences add to your day-to-day stress and frustration, and as you continue to struggle, you become discouraged, overwhelmed, and depressed. This only adds to the difficulties you have in getting things done.

The goal then of time and task management skills is to help you get more done with the time you have and feel less stressed and frustrated in the process. Who couldn't use skills like that?

Skill: Increase Time and Task Awareness

The first step in learning to manage time and tasks is to know what you do with your time and the amount of time these activities and tasks typically take. Use the Time and Task Awareness Log to record these activities.

Instructions

1. Select a day and a window of time, perhaps from when you awaken to lunch, or for a period of time (for example, 9:00 a.m. to 12:00 p.m.). In the log, write what you plan to do and estimate how long you think the task will take, and when you plan to start the task.

2. After you complete the activity or task, write in the log how long the task actually took to complete and the actual time you started the task. Try this for a few days to get a good sense of where your time goes.

Time and Task Awareness Log

Activity or Task	Estimated Time to Complete	Scheduled Time to Start	Actual Time Completed	Actual Time Started
Outline monthly progress report.	30 minutes	1:30 p.m.	45 minutes	2:15 p.m.

Now that you've completed a few days of recording with the log, calculate your Time-to-Task Ratio (TTR) for each task: [Actual Time to Complete] – [Estimated Time to Complete] ÷ [Estimated Time to Complete] x 100%. From the example, 45 – 30 ÷ 30 x 100% = +50%. Next, average these ratios to calculate the average Time-to-Task Ratio (TTR).

If your TTR average is 0%, then you're a perfect time-to-task estimator. If your TTR average is a (+) number, then you tend to *underestimate* the amount of time to complete tasks. Try adding this average TTR percent to your time estimates. For example, if your average TTR is +25%, add 10 minutes to your initial estimate of 40 minutes. If your TTR average is a (–) number, then you tend to *overestimate* the amount of time to complete tasks. Try subtracting this average TTR percent from your time estimates. For example, if your average TTR is -10%, then subtract 4 minutes from your initial estimate of 40 minutes.

Next, calculate (in minutes) your Time-to-Start Factor (TSF) for each task: [Scheduled Time to Start] – [Actual Time Started]. From the example 1:30 p.m. – 2:15 p.m. = -45 minutes. Now average these numbers to calculate the average Time-to-Start Ratio (TSF). If your TSF is 0, then you tend to start tasks immediately without even a moment of delay. Great job! If your TSF is a negative (-) number, then you tend to delay or procrastinate starting tasks. Try some of the skills in this chapter to decrease your TSF and procrastinate less.

Describe what you learned. How good are you at estimating the amount of time tasks take? Do you tend to procrastinate or are you quick to start and complete tasks? As you paid attention to what you do and when you start, what did you notice when you delayed starting?

_____

_____

_____

_____

_____

_____

Skill: Manage Time

Who hasn't said, "Wow, the time got away from me." But if time too often gets away from you, then you can suffer short- and long-term consequences: missed appointments, missed deadlines, missed opportunities.

In the previous skill, you learned something about your ability to estimate how much time it takes you to complete typical tasks. It helps to think of tasks in terms of time because you can better schedule tasks in your calendar if you know about how much time tasks will take. If you tend to underestimate the time tasks take, try the following:

- **Build a bit of wiggle room into your schedule.** Schedule thirty to sixty minutes before lunch and after lunch to accommodate surprises. For example, you encounter unexpected traffic, or your boss drops an unscheduled meeting into your calendar, or you realize that you need something to complete the project and it will take time to get it. A little wiggle room is a life saver.

- **Use a timer.** If you tend to get distracted, a timer is a great way to stay on track. Set a timer for five or ten minutes before you start a task. When the timer sounds, ask yourself, "Am I still working on the task I started when I set the timer?" If the answer is yes, then reset the timer and resume working on the task. If the answer is no, then go back to the original task and set the timer again. This way, you only lose five or ten minutes rather than forty minutes working on tasks that you didn't intend to work on initially.

- **Improve your time awareness**. If you tend to float from moment to moment with little awareness of time passing, try this simple game to increase your time awareness as well as improve your ability to estimate time. As you go through the day, stop and ask yourself what time you think it is. For example, if it was 10:00 a.m. the last time you looked at a clock, as you go through the day, stop and estimate the time and then check the clock. With practice, you'll improve your ability to estimate the time of day pretty accurately.

A second way to improve your time awareness is to use the Estimate Time Accurately Log.

Instructions

1. For several weeks, estimate and record how much time you think a task will take, then rate and record how confident you are that estimate is correct.

2. After you complete the task, record how much time it actually took you to complete the task. With practice, you'll notice that your confidence in your ability to estimate time-to-task increases as your ability to estimate time-to-task accurately improves.

Estimate Time Accurately Log			
Task	Estimated Time (mins.)	Confidence in Estimate (0–100%)	Actual Time (mins.)
File completed reports.	30 minutes	50%	45 minutes

Skill: Practice Strategic Time Management

If you were stranded on an island with only a backpack of food, you'd likely plan what, how much, and when to eat the meager rations you have. It helps to think of time this way. It's a limited resource that is important for you to ration thoughtfully. To practice strategic time management, consider the following:

- What time in the day are you most rested and focused? What more demanding tasks can you schedule then?

- Are there limited times of the day that you can do this task (for example, call the dentist's office)? What could you do now and then set aside the next step until this time that's limited?

- Is this a task that you can do at the same time as you work on another task (for example, what task could you do while you're on hold, what task could you do while you're waiting for your dental appointment)?

- Is it best to focus only on this task or can you do this task while you do another task?

- Can you delegate this task to someone?

- If you do this task now, will you sleep better tonight?

- If you require something to start this task, when could you get it and how?

Try strategic time management for one week. Remember, time is a resource and you're learning to manage that resource by making smart choices with your time given the ins and outs of your day-to-day life. Use what you learned in the Increase Time and Task Awareness skill to estimate accurately the amount of time any task will take. However, when working on a task or project that you've not done before, build in a little more time for your learning curve.

Describe what you learned after a week of strategic time management. Were there any surprises about the decisions you made with your time, and what were they? Which time management strategy worked best for you? Which time management strategy worked least well, and why?

_____

_____

_____

_____

_____

_____

Skill: Break Down Tasks

When you're anxious, depressed, or simply overwhelmed by the many things you have to do, it's harder to get things done. You convince yourself that you'll do it later when you have more energy, or when you're less stressed. As you put things off, your anxiety builds, your mood crashes, and you feel more and more overwhelmed. Now, it feels impossible to start a project, even a small one, much less finish it. To get things moving, it helps to break a big project into smaller projects or steps.

Instructions

1. Think of a project or task that you're putting off starting. It could be a school project, home project, or anything else.

2. Ask yourself, "How many parts can I divide this task into?" Then, divide the task or project into as many small steps as you can think of.

3. Look at each step. Rate how confident (0 to 100 percent, where 100 percent is completely confident) you are that you could start and complete the step as you described it. Try for a confidence level of 90 percent or greater. If you feel less than 90 percent, break that small step into a couple of smaller steps. To help rate your confidence level, ask yourself:

   - How long did it take me to complete similar tasks in the past?

   - How long did it take me to complete similar tasks when under pressure?

   - How long did it take me to complete similar tasks when I was working efficiently?

   - How long does it take a friend or coworker to complete similar tasks?

4. Keep breaking down each step until you have steps that you're very confident (90 percent or greater) that you can start and complete.

Skill: Prioritize Tasks

You've likely heard that a powerful way to get more done is to prioritize tasks before you start to work on them. There are several advantages to prioritizing tasks:

- **Increased productivity:** Completing the most important tasks first has the greatest impact on your productivity. They're important tasks for a reason.

- **Decreased stress and worry:** As you complete the important tasks first, you'll feel less worried about missing important deadlines. Less worry and anxiety will improve your ability to concentrate and thereby work efficiently.

- **You'll know when you're procrastinating:** If you're working on less important tasks when you haven't started or completed more important tasks, then you're procrastinating. You'll learn other skills in this chapter to procrastinate less, but in order to stop procrastinating, it's essential to know when you're doing it.

The ABC method is a simple way to prioritize tasks into three categories relative to importance:

- *A-tasks:* These tasks are typically urgent tasks with deadlines and you complete these first before you start B-tasks or C-tasks. Most A-tasks are "complete by the end of the day" tasks or within twenty-four hours, such as when your boss asks you to create an agenda for the meeting later that day or when it's important to meet with a coworker before they leave for the day.

- *B-tasks:* These tasks aren't necessarily associated with a deadline but are important to complete relatively soon, such as organizing an office party or preparing for a meeting next week. You complete these tasks usually within a week or two.

- *C-tasks:* These tasks are the least important tasks in your schedule, such as filing paperwork or straightening your desk.

A-Task Tips

If an A-task is a big project that you can't complete in a day, break down the task into subtasks and use numbers to prioritize those, such as A1, A2, A3. However, always work on

A-tasks before B-tasks or C-tasks even if the A task is an A33 because even an A33 task is more important than a B-task.

Work on A-tasks during your best times of the day. For some people, that's first thing in the morning. For other people, it's before lunch. Watch for a tendency to work on A-tasks later in the day, however. You may be procrastinating.

B-Task Tips

If you have multiple B-tasks, use numbers to prioritize them as well, such as B1, B2, B3. This will help you focus on the most important B-task before starting the next one. Because A-tasks are the most important to complete, you'll likely want to do those tasks yourself, so consider delegating B-tasks.

C-Task Tips

You may be able to delegate C-tasks too, but C-tasks can be great tasks to complete when you have a spare minute or two, such as while waiting to pick up your child or waiting for everyone to arrive for a meeting. However, this requires some planning, so take a look at your schedule and your list of C-tasks and jot down which C-task to do in spare moments.

Skill: Plan Ahead

A few minutes at the end of the day (or at the beginning of the day, if you prefer) can create some momentum to the next day and is a great way to reward yourself for what you've completed. To help with this, use the Plan Ahead Schedule.

Instructions

1. Set aside a few minutes at the end of the day to plan for the next day.

2. Review what you completed for the day and create a to-do list for the next day.

3. Prioritize these tasks.

Plan Ahead Schedule				
Time	Task or Activity (be specific)	A	B	C
2:00 p.m.	Call Janice and schedule team meeting for next week.	✓		
6:00 a.m.				
7:00 a.m.				
8:00 a.m.				
9:00 a.m.				
10:00 a.m.				
11:00 a.m.				
12:00 p.m.				
1:00 p.m.				
2:00 p.m.				
3:00 p.m.				
4:00 p.m.				
5:00 p.m.				
6:00 p.m.				
7:00 p.m.				
8:00 p.m.				
9:00 p.m.				
10:00 p.m.				
11:00 p.m.				
12:00 a.m.				

Skill: Do It Now

Many times, we talk ourselves into not doing something: I'm too tired today. I don't have time. Or an all-time favorite: I'll do it later. Perhaps you did it later or perhaps you didn't. A little of this "do-it-later" attitude isn't likely to create big problems in your life. But if you have a habitual pattern of putting off until later what would be in your best interest to do now, and this pattern results in significant short- and long-term consequences for you (more stress or unhappiness, lost jobs or relationships), then you may struggle with the biggest obstacle to effective time and task management: a do-it-later attitude. There are three ingredients to any plan to overcome procrastination and the do-it-later attitude that fuels it:

- **Awareness:** You can't overcome procrastination if you're unaware that you're doing it. To increase your awareness, set a timer for ten minutes. When it sounds, ask yourself, "Have I started work on the task?" If the answer is yes, then reset the timer and continue to work. If the answer is no, then reset the timer and start. Also, remember the ABC priority system? If you have A-tasks and you're working on B- or C-tasks, or you have B-tasks and you're working on C-tasks, then you're procrastinating.

- **Do-it-now attitude:** Procrastination is avoidance: Avoiding tasks that make you anxious or bring you down. Avoiding tasks that take a lot of mental effort. Avoiding tasks that you know will take a lot of time because you believe that you must do them perfectly. Regardless of the reasons that you procrastinate, it tends to begin with one or more "permission to do it later" thoughts:

  - I can't start until I have enough time to finish the entire task.

  - I'll start after I do more research.

  - I'll wait until I know I can do this.

  - I'll start when I have more energy.

  - I have to be certain I know how to do this before I start.

  Try countering your *do-it-later* thoughts with *do-it-now* thoughts. For example, to the thought, "I'll do it when I have more time," counter it with something like, "You don't know if you'll have more time later. Do some work now with the time that you have now."

- **Action in the face of discomfort:** If you procrastinate, it's because you've made the decision to avoid discomfort (anxiety, fatigue, sadness, boredom, or guilt) rather than moving a task or project ahead in the face of it. To overcome procrastination, it's essential that you act in the face of discomfort like this. To increase your willingness to act in the face of discomfort, ask yourself:

  - What do I lose or risk if I continue to procrastinate?

  - What will I gain (free time, positive relationships, success) if I start now?

  - What will I gain if I finish the task?

To help overcome procrastination, look at the example worksheet and then use the Do-It-Now Worksheet to practice this skill.

Instructions

1. Set aside a few minutes and consider what tasks you're putting off starting. Be honest with yourself. If you have a to-do list, scan that and identify a task that has been sitting on the list for a long time. Write the task in the space on the worksheet.

2. In the Permission to Put It Off Attitude section, write what you're telling yourself that makes procrastinating okay enough that you are willing to put off starting.

3. In the Lose section, write what you lose in the short and long term by putting it off. Remember, short-term consequences can be unpleasant feelings (guilt that you disappointed someone, frustration with yourself about a missed deadline). Long-term consequences are the consequences you've experienced in the past (missed opportunity, upset coworker, lost friendship) that could happen again if you procrastinate.

4. In the Do-It-Now Attitude section, write what you could tell yourself that would make it okay to start the task now. At times you'll write what you know is the truth, such as "I tell myself that I'll do it when I have more time, but I don't really know if I'll have more time later," and follow it with a statement that encourages you to start now regardless of the reasons you give yourself to put off starting.

5. In the Gain section, write what you'll gain if you start the task now. At times, what you gain is less of something (less guilt, less stress, less disappointment). At other

times, what you gain is more of something (more time to do fun things, stronger friendships, greater self-confidence).

6. Last, in the Plan section, write your plan. What skills or strategies might you use to start now and stay on track? Include in your plan ways to remind yourself to do it now (timers, notes). Also, write what you'll gain by doing it now as well as what you'll say to those pesky thoughts you've identified that give you permission to put off starting the task now.

Do-It-Now Worksheet	
Awareness What am I putting off?	
Preparing my presentation for the team meeting on Friday.	
Permission to Put It Off Attitude What am I telling myself that makes it okay to put it off?	**Do-It-Now Attitude** What could I tell myself that makes it okay to start now?
I'll do it when I have more time.	You don't know if you'll have more time later. Do some work now with the time that you have now.
Lose What do I lose if I continue to put this off?	**Gain** What do I gain if I do it now?
More guilt, stress, and frustration with myself because I didn't have enough time to do a good job.	Time to do something fun without worrying whether I'll have time to finish the presentation.
Plan What's my plan to face discomfort and do it now?	
I'll use a timer to help me start and stay on track. I'll tape a note on my computer, "Are you working on your presentation or are you procrastinating?" I'll watch for my favorite do-it-later thought, "I'll do it when I have more time," and counter it with, "You don't know if you'll have more time later. Do some work now with the time you have now." I'll also remind myself of what I gain by starting, which is more time to spend with my kids, as well as what I lose if I continue to procrastinate: stress, frustration, and guilt.	

Do-It-Now Worksheet

Awareness
What am I putting off?

Permission to Put It Off Attitude	Do-It-Now Attitude
What am I telling myself that makes it okay to put it off?	What could I tell myself that makes it okay to start now?

Lose	Gain
What do I lose if I continue to put this off?	What do I gain if I do it now?

Plan
What's my plan to face discomfort and do it now?

Skill: Solve Problems

When you're anxious, depressed, hopeless, stressed, or simply overwhelmed, little problems can feel huge. You may feel paralyzed and unable to think clearly about the problem or how to solve it. That's when this problem-solving skill can help the most. Use the Solve Problems Worksheet to help you feel more calm, capable, and hopeful.

Instructions

1. Define the problem.

2. Brainstorm potential solutions that might help.

3. Consider the advantages and disadvantages of each potential solution.

4. Rank potential solutions in terms of priority on a scale of 1 to 4 (1 = most likely to help).

5. Select the #1 rank solution and plan how you'll implement it. The best solution is the one most likely to work and least likely to cause you more problems. There is seldom a perfect solution to a problem, but there are many good solutions that can help and not make things worse. Remember, you can't know whether a solution will work until you try it.

6. Review how well the solution worked. To do this, imagine a target. If you hit the bull's-eye, then your solution worked great. This means you got what you wanted *and* it didn't create other problems for you.

7. Decide the next step. If the solution hit the target but wasn't a bull's-eye, this means you'll want to modify the solution a little. If the solution missed the target completely, this means it didn't work at all or, worse yet, created more problems for you. Select the next (#2 rank) solution.

Solve Problems Worksheet

Problem:

Brainstorm potential solutions

Solution 1:	
Solution 2:	
Solution 3:	
Solution 4:	

List the advantages and disadvantages of each potential solution

Solution 1: Rank _____	
Advantages:	
Disadvantages:	
Solution 2: Rank _____	
Advantages:	
Disadvantages:	

Solution 3: Rank _____	
Advantages:	
Disadvantages:	
Solution 4: Rank _____	
Advantages:	
Disadvantages:	

Review advantages and disadvantages of each solution and rank in priority (1–4):

Plan how you'll implement the rank #1 solution:	
When and Where	
Steps	1. _____ 2. _____ 3. _____ 4. _____

Review how well solution worked and decide the next step:

You can apply this problem-solving skill to most problems, including social problems, such as a boss who repeatedly asks you to work weekends or a friend who is chronically late. As you might guess, many of the solutions to social problems involve the interpersonal effectiveness skills you learned in the previous chapter.

Wrap Up

Time and task management skills can improve your effectiveness in life. With these skills, you'll get more done and more quickly with the time you have. Not only that, but you'll also feel less overwhelmed and frustrated as you move through your to-do list.

In the next chapter, you'll learn a systematic way to build your tolerance to intense negative feelings. With greater emotion tolerance, your emotional responses begin to operate like the emotional responses of other people. You'll feel less intensely anxious, depressed, guilty, or frustrated by life events and your emotional system will recover more quickly from these events. That's when life gets easier.

CHAPTER 7

Emotion Exposure Skills

Perhaps the primary reason you're reading this workbook is that you want to learn skills to feel less anxious, depressed, or guilty, and so far you've learned skills to do this. Skills to regulate the intensity of these negative emotions are great, but these skills don't always decrease their persistence over time. What's the point, you might ask, of feeling less anxious or depressed if you continue to feel this level—although lower—all the time? It's a great point, and emotion exposure skills help with that.

Emotion exposure skills are a set of behavioral strategies that build your tolerance to negative emotions and, as a result, decrease the intensity *and* persistence of these feelings (Barlow, Allen, and Choate 2016). Emotion exposure skills are *inside skills* because they target the internal features of emotions: thoughts and physical sensations.

Why Are Emotion Exposure Skills Important?

Through emotion exposure skills, you'll learn that you can tolerate negative emotions, such as anxiety, sadness, guilt, or shame. As you learn that you can tolerate negative emotions, you'll experience unexpected and even counterintuitive benefits (Tompkins 2021) such as:

- **Learning that you can tolerate negative emotions dampens their intensity over time.** Although facing negative emotions increases the emotion in the short term, the intensity of negative emotions decreases over time. It's counterintuitive, but it works.

- **Learning that you can tolerate negative emotions dampens their persistence over time.** Repeatedly facing negative emotions builds an emotional system that returns to baseline more quickly. This means that negative emotional responses don't persist but dampen in a few minutes as normal emotional responses do.

- **Learning that you can tolerate negative emotions builds confidence.** Negative emotions are part of life's challenges. Repeatedly facing negative emotions increases confidence that you can handle the difficulties of life and the feelings that accompany them.

How Emotion Exposure Works

To understand how emotion exposure skills build emotion tolerance, consider how you'd go about building your tolerance to cold showers. You would likely repeatedly take cold showers, perhaps extending the length of the shower over time. Although repeated cold showers doesn't increase the temperature of the water, it does increase your confidence that you can tolerate a cold temperature. With greater confidence, you'll dread cold showers less. With less dread, you'll avoid cold showers less. But here's the real payoff—and it's a bit of a paradox—as you repeatedly take cold showers, your experience of cold showers changes too. The showers begin to feel tolerable, certainly more tolerable than how intolerable they felt at first. This paradox works with negative emotions too. Approaching rather than avoiding negative emotions dampens the intensity of these emotions over time.

Three emotion exposure skills can build emotion tolerance:

- **Resist emotion-driven action urges.** These are subtle actions that dampen negative emotions when you cannot avoid or leave a situation. For example, you might keep your hands in your pockets to avoid feeling anxious that someone will think you're weird if they see that your hands are trembling, or you keep to yourself because you believe that you lack the energy to speak to anyone.

- **Approach and remain in situations that evoke negative feelings.** These are situation emotion exposures. You might avoid the negative feelings that arise when you interact with certain objects, participate in certain activities, or enter certain situations. For example, you might avoid attending a party because you're worried about what people might think about you, or you might avoid attending a work party because you feel guilty about enjoying yourself when you haven't finished your work.

- **Approach and stay with thoughts and images that evoke negative feelings.** These are thought exposures. Although you're not at the party yet, thoughts that you might say something stupid loom large in your mind. You might then distract yourself to avoid thinking about the party, but as you do this you can't think about anything else. Similarly, if you're depressed about a recent breakup, you might remember the look on the face of your ex when he told you that he wanted a divorce. This image may cause you to feel intensely guilty and depressed because you believe it's all your fault that your ex left.

To benefit fully from emotion exposures, it's essential that you practice the same emotion exposure repeatedly until your discomfort decreases to 50 percent or more of the maximum or peak of your distress. Set aside at least thirty to forty minutes each day to practice and practice at least three or four times a week. This is quite a commitment, but with consistent and adequate practice for several weeks, your life will open again as you reverse years of avoiding and fleeing from negative feelings.

Prepare and Plan Emotion Exposures

Effective emotion exposures take planning, as well as preparing yourself to approach intense negative feelings that you've likely spent many years avoiding. Here's how to plan:

Instructions

1. Identify urges, thoughts, and physical sensations that are part of your negative feelings.

2. Connect with the values you'll use to motivate yourself to face negative feelings.

3. FACE the negative feelings to benefit fully from each emotion exposure.

4. Build a resist emotion-driven action plan.

5. Build an emotion exposure menu.

Regardless of the type of exposure you do, use the Emotion Exposure Planning Worksheet to set up and record the practice and, most importantly, what you learned in the process. Tracking your emotion exposure practice in this way increases your willingness to try future practices because you learn that you can tolerate these intense feelings.

Skill: Identify Features of Negative Feelings

Emotion exposures can be difficult, but with a little preparation and planning, you can get the most out of each one. The first step is to identify the action urges, thoughts, images, memories, and physical sensations that are part of your intense negative feelings.

For example, Miles, who feels intensely anxious in social situations, identified:

- *Action urges:* Hands in my pockets; avoid looking at people; make excuses to leave early.

- *Thoughts, images, memories:* Thoughts about saying something stupid; image of people asking about my trembling hands; memory of nearly having a panic attack last year.

- *Physical sensations:* Hands shaking; sweating; blushing.

Julie, who is depressed and often feels intensely guilty too, identified:

- *Action urges:* Not speaking to my married friends; checking social media to see what Bob's doing; going to bed.

- *Thoughts, images, memories:* Memory of Bob telling me he wanted a divorce; image of Bob leaving the house for last time; thoughts that it's my fault he left.

- *Physical sensations:* Heaviness; tiredness; difficulty concentrating; tearful.

Instructions

1. Take a few minutes and think back over the past week or two. What action urges arose that you avoided?

2. What thoughts, images, or memories triggered intense negative emotions, such as anxiety, fear, sadness, guilt, or shame?

3. Over the next few weeks, add to the worksheet as you identify new urges, thoughts, or sensations.

Emotion Exposure Planning Worksheet	
Action Urges	
Thoughts, Images, Memories	
Physical Sensations	

Skill: Connect with Your Values

There is likely no skill in this workbook more challenging than emotion exposure; therefore, it's essential that you remain motivated as you face uncomfortable feelings.

Instructions

1. Review the value-action statements you developed in chapter 1. Write those value-action words, actions and statements in the Value-Action Statements Worksheet. You'll use those during the emotion exposure practice that follows. Or write new value-action statements and enter those in the worksheet.

2. Now, before you practice one of the emotion exposure skills, close your eyes and repeat the value-action statement to yourself several times. Imagine yourself doing the value action. Then, as you start the value action, repeat the value-action statement under your breath, as if you're talking yourself through it.

Value-Action Statements Worksheet

Value Word:	Relationships
Value Action:	Resolve conflicts.
Value-Action Statement:	In order to strengthen and deepen my relationships, I will call Irma and apologize even though I'm worried that she'll be upset with me.
Value Word:	
Value Action:	
Value-Action Statement:	
Value Word:	
Value Action:	
Value-Action Statement:	

Skill: FACE Negative Emotions

For the full benefit of emotion exposures, it's important that you practice emotion exposures correctly. Follow these steps to FACE negative emotions.

Instructions

1. **F**ace your negative feeling. Over the years, you've fallen into a pattern or habit of turning away from negative feelings. Learning to face your negative feelings is essential if you're to build tolerance to them.

2. **A**nchor to the present moment. Anchoring to the present moment means feeling what's happening now. In this way, you learn that you have nothing to fear from feeling your feelings, and that you can handle these feelings as they come and go. Review the meditation skills that you learned in chapter 3. Prior to each emotion exposure, spend a few minutes in a mindful attitude to prepare yourself for the feelings to come.

3. **C**heck or resist your emotion-driven actions. Resist the subtle ways you avoid, lessen, or attempt to control negative feelings. During an emotion exposure, don't say prayers or affirmations, distract yourself, visualize positive outcomes, or do anything that takes you away from the feeling. In other words, resist urges to act but don't resist the feeling itself. Emotion-driven actions only get in the way of you learning that you can tolerate unpleasant negative feelings.

4. **E**ndure the negative feelings. It's essential that you endure negative feelings until they decrease on their own, without trying to control these feelings in any way. If you have trouble enduring your feelings, drop down to a less challenging item in the emotion exposure menu (you'll learn about the menu later in this chapter) or add easier menu items and start there.

Skill: Resist and Delay Emotion-Driven Actions

A great way to build emotion tolerance is to resist the emotion-driven actions you use to escape, decrease, or control negative emotions. Each time you use an emotion-driven action, you chip away at the confidence in your emotion tolerance that you're working to build.

Normal and natural emotions come and go, rise and fall. The entire process usually takes five minutes or less. Therefore, when something triggers a negative emotion, the key is to wait out the feeling. As the negative feeling decreases, the intensity of the action urge decreases too. Use the Emotion-Driven Action Delay Log to practice this skill.

Instructions

1. List the emotion-driven actions you plan to resist.

2. Set a delay goal (in minutes). This is the length of time that you commit to resisting the action urge. Set a delay time that you're confident (0 to 100 percent, where 100 percent is completely confident) you can successfully complete. Try for a confidence level of 85 percent or higher. For example, if you're 60 percent confident you can delay an emotion-driven action for ten minutes, set a shorter time until you're in the 85 to 90 percent confidence range. Write this time in *T1* and the confidence level in *CL*.

3. Write a *value-action statement* to increase your willingness to delay. For example, if relationships are an important value and you repeatedly ask your partner for reassurance, which often leads to arguments, your value-action statement might read, "In order to strengthen and deepen my marriage, I will resist asking my partner for reassurance when I'm anxious about my health."

4. Now, repeat the value-action statement to yourself as you resist and FACE the action urge. Feel free to do something while you wait for the intensity of the action urge to decrease. It's okay to do something else as long as it helps you resist the emotion-driven action.

5. At the end of your delay goal, repeat the process. Ask yourself how much longer you can delay. Again, select a delay goal that you're confident (greater than 85 percent) you can complete. This is *T2*. Write this time and the confidence level (*CL*) in the log.

6. Again, repeat your value-action statement and FACE the action urge, then engage in an alternative activity as long as you don't use it to feel less uncomfortable.

7. Repeat steps 4 and 5 as long as you feel the action urge.

Emotion-Driven Action Delay Log										
Emotion-Driven Action	Delay Time and Confidence Level									
	T1	CL	T2	CL	T3	CL	T4	CL	T5	CL

Describe what you observed as you resisted emotion-driven actions. Did the feelings rise and fall? Did you learn anything about your negative feelings that surprised you?

_____

_____

_____

_____

_____

Situation Emotion Exposure

An emotion exposure practice menu provides a road map for emotion exposure practices. You'll have a menu for each type of exposure you practice: situations, thoughts, and physical sensations. As you think through possible menu items for situation emotion exposures, consider the following variables that influence negative feelings:

- *Proximity* to an object or situation can influence the intensity of your negative feelings. For Lucas, who was afraid of heights, the distance to a ledge or an overlook influenced his anxiety. Lucas added menu items such as standing ten feet, five feet, and one foot away from a balcony.

- *Time* spent in a situation or near an object can influence the intensity of your negative feelings. Miles, for example, worried that others would notice his hands shaking and think that he was weird, and therefore he kept his hands in his pockets when around people. Miles added menu items such as ten minutes, five minutes, and one minute with hands out of his pockets when interacting with people.

- *Size, degree, or importance* can influence the intensity of your negative feelings too. For example, Miles was more anxious when interacting with important people like his boss, or with people he didn't know well.

Skill: Build a Situation Emotion Exposure Practice Menu

To build a situation emotion exposure menu, use the Emotion Exposure Menu Planner.

Instructions

1. **Select practice situations.** Think about the situations that trigger negative feelings. Describe each situation in as specific and detailed a way as you can. Consider situations that you avoid or situations that trigger emotion-driven actions, such as checking, distracting, or seeking reassurance from others. Add a few over-the-top items, such as Miles intentionally shaking his hands a little when speaking with people.

2. **Identify emotion-driven actions.** Identify the typical emotion-driven actions you use to avoid or control the intensity of your negative feelings. Write these in the *Emotion-Driven Actions* column.

3. **Identify alternative actions.** To get the most out of every emotion exposure practice, it's essential that you resist doing any emotion-driven actions during an emotion exposure. In the *Alternative Action* column, add the alternative actions you'll practice during the emotion exposure. For example, when Emily rides an escalator, she closes her eyes and leans away from the handrail. Emily turned these emotion-driven actions into alternative actions, such as keeping her eyes open and leaning toward the handrail a little.

4. **Rank practice situations.** Rank the situations on a scale of 0 to 100 based on the intensity of the emotion you predict you'll feel if you engage in the situation or activity completely without doing any emotion-driven actions. If two practice situations feel as if they would be equally difficult, ask yourself which you would do first. You'll likely select the one that's a little easier. Place that below the other one on your practice menu. Rate each situation from 0 to 100 and write these numbers in the *Rank* column.

	Emotion Exposure Menu Planner		
Rank	Practice Situation	Emotion-Driven Actions	Alternative Actions
70	Ride up escalator.	Close eyes or look away. Lean away from handrail.	Keep eyes open. Lean toward handrail a little.

Skill: Practice Situation Emotion Exposure

Now that you've created your emotion exposure menu, it's time to practice the first emotion exposure. Prior to the emotion exposure, look at the example worksheet and then complete the first half of the Emotion Exposure Practice Log. Remember, the goal of emotion exposure is for you to learn something that you may not believe deep down: that you can tolerate the negative emotions that arise while you face the feelings in the present moment. To help with this new learning, it's important to track what you've learned in previous exposures and what you think, particularly what you expect to happen, and what you want to remember during the upcoming exposure.

Instructions

1. Select a situation from the practice menu. You can begin with any menu item you wish, as long as you're confident (85 percent or greater) that you can resist any action urges that arise. Engaging in action urges during any emotion exposure dilutes the benefit of the exposure and your hard work.

2. Review the emotion-driven actions you'll resist for that exposure and the alternative actions you'll do. Remember, if you're doing alternative actions, you're less likely to do emotion-driven actions. Not only that, but doing alternative actions also gives a boost to the exposures you do.

3. If you haven't written a *value-action statement* for this emotion practice, write one now and repeat it to yourself a few times. For example, if professional achievement is an important value to you and your fear of having a panic attack on the subway prevents you from getting to work, your value-action statement might read, "In order to achieve my professional goals and be as successful as I know I can be, I will face my fear and ride the subway."

4. Now, repeat the value-action statement to yourself as you FACE your negative feeling. Once you've anchored to your breath, open your attention to include the negative feeling. You may feel a bit anxious as you anticipate stepping into feelings you've likely avoided for many months and perhaps years. This is natural and part of the process of building emotion tolerance. Observe your negative feelings without judging or analyzing them. Stay with the feelings and watch them in the moment. Accept them and

remind yourself that they come and go. Don't forget to practice the alternative actions and resist emotion-driven actions.

5. Repeat step 4 until your discomfort decreases to 50 percent or less of the maximum or peak of your distress. It's essential that you repeat emotion exposures within a period of time, if you can, to experience the benefit. For example, ride the subway six times (or more), one ride after another.

6. At the end of each situation emotion exposure, complete the bottom half of the log. It's essential that you spend some time reflecting on what you learned from every emotion exposure you complete. Don't forget to describe what you learned that was helpful. Did what you expected to happen occur? For example, if you expected that you wouldn't enjoy yourself at all during lunch with friends, did that happen or not? And most important, were you able to tolerate the negative feeling?

Emotion Exposure Practice Log

Emotion Exposure Task: Walk Boomer for ten minutes in the morning and smile at everyone I pass.

Prior Learning to Remember for This Practice

Last time I did this exposure, I saw about seven people with their dogs. Every person I smiled at smiled back and several women stopped to chat with me. I felt much better at the end of the walk. Usually walking Boomer is a drudge, but last time, I enjoyed it more and especially enjoyed chatting with the women I met.

Before Emotion Exposure Practice

Rate anticipatory discomfort level (0–10):	4
Rate confidence you can tolerate discomfort for length of exposure (0–100%):	70%

What are you expecting? I won't have the energy to speak to people who want to speak with me. I'm much more tired than the last time I did this.

What physical sensations are you feeling? Some trouble concentrating, heavy, tired, and a little tense.

What action urges are you feeling and what emotion-driven actions will you resist?

I'm thinking of not going this morning. I know avoiding is my MO, so I'm going to go, but I'm thinking up excuses to tell my therapist for why I bailed out.

After Emotion Exposure Practice

Length of practice (mins.):	15 min
Maximum discomfort level during practice (0–10):	5
Discomfort level at end of practice (0–10):	2
Re-rate confidence you can tolerate discomfort for length of exposure (0–100%):	80%

What did you learn?

I learned again that I can handle the guilty feelings I have when I do something good or fun for myself. I also learned that just because I'm having trouble concentrating or if I feel tired, I can still walk Boomer. And once I smile at someone and talk with them, I start to feel much better pretty quickly. I guess the bottom line is to tolerate the guilt I feel so that I can take care of myself. It's okay. Just because I enjoy myself doesn't make me a bad mother.

Emotion Exposure Practice Log

Emotion Exposure Task:

Prior Learning to Remember for This Practice

Before Emotion Exposure Practice

Rate anticipatory discomfort level (0–10):	
Rate confidence you can tolerate discomfort for length of exposure (0–100%):	
What are you expecting?	
What physical sensations are you feeling?	
What action urges are you feeling and what emotion-driven actions will you resist?	

After Emotion Exposure Practice

Length of practice (mins.):	
Maximum discomfort level during practice (0–10):	
Discomfort level at end of practice (0–10):	
Re-rate confidence you can tolerate discomfort for length of exposure (0–100%):	

What did you learn?

Thought Emotion Exposure

Thought emotion exposure is the process of turning toward rather than away from the thoughts, memories, and images that fuel your negative feelings. Through the emotion exposure process, these negative cognitions become less frequent, less intense, and less important. You'll use the same approach and strategies you learned for situation emotion exposures, including building a practice menu.

Skill: Build a Thought Emotion Exposure Practice Menu

To create a thought exposure menu, you'll use the Emotion Exposure Menu Planner that you already filled out.

Instructions

1. Create a scenario for each menu item. Try to include as much detail in the scenarios as possible and as if it's happening to you now.

2. Write the scenario in the first person and include as many of your thoughts and feelings as you can. Include also the unpleasant physical sensations that arise and the urges you have to avoid them.

For example, Lucas, who is afraid of heights, developed several menu items in which he imagined standing on the edge of the step in a stairwell and looking down to the landing below. In one menu item, he imagined feeling dizzy and light-headed as he struggled to keep his balance on the stair. He imagined that his body was trembling and that his knees were shaking as he tipped forward, feeling as if he was about to fall down the stairs. He created an even scarier menu item in which he imagined himself actually falling down the stairs, overcome with dizziness, unable to control his body, tipping forward and tumbling down the stairs, one after another, powerless to stop. Lucas created a menu with six separate scenes—each scene a menu item—from the least scary to most scary. Scenes lowest in distress included riding the escalator while he felt light-headed or driving on certain stretches of freeway waiting for the dizziness to strike. Here's one of the scenarios Lucas wrote:

I'm on the landing in the stairwell at work. I'm stepping off the landing to the first step when the dizziness hits me. I grab for the handrail, but I can't seem to find it because I'm so dizzy. My legs and hands are trembling. I try to lean back from the edge, but the dizziness overwhelms me and I can't control my body. I feel myself beginning to tip forward. I try desperately to lean away from the step, but I'm so confused that I lean forward. I begin to feel myself, falling. I'm trying to stop but I can't. I feel completely out of control as I slowly tip forward. I'm in slow motion as I watch myself fall. I stretch out my hands to protect myself, but the fear paralyzes me. I can't move my arms. I slowly begin to topple like a tree, slowly falling toward the steps below.

Julie developed several menu scenarios. The easiest scenario was sitting in the living room while her kids were in school. She described the intense feelings of loneliness and guilt, as well as thoughts that she'd ruined her kids' lives because of the divorce. She wrote a moderately intense scenario in which she was at a party and enjoying herself, but feeling intensely guilty that she didn't deserve to be happy because of what she had done to cause the divorce. In the most intensely uncomfortable scenario, Julie imagined her ex-husband telling her that he wants a divorce because she's been a bad spouse and mother. Julie described that she felt "punched in the gut" and intensely guilty and depressed as she saw the look of disgust on her ex-husband's face and how he shook his head and walked away. She described trouble focusing and extreme heaviness in her body in that moment. Here's one of the scenarios that Julie wrote:

I'm hanging out with Cindy in the living room. We're scrapbooking and having a great time. I haven't enjoyed myself this much in many months. I'm smiling and laughing. I then start to think about my kids. I think that only a horrible mother would choose to have fun when her kids have been so deeply affected by the divorce. I'm feeling intensely guilty. I keep thinking that I've ruined their lives and that it's all my fault. I know that if I had been a better spouse, my husband wouldn't have left me. It's so selfish of me to have fun with Cindy while my kids are suffering. I'm a horrible mother, a horrible person, and I deserve every bad thing that's happened to me.

Skill: Practice Thought Emotion Exposure

Now that you've created a menu in which each of the scenarios you wrote is a menu item, it's time to practice thought emotion exposures. To practice thought emotion exposures, refer to your completed Emotion Exposure Menu Planner and fill in the Emotion Exposure Practice Log.

Instructions

1. Select a scenario that you completed earlier. You can begin with any menu item you wish, as long as you're confident (85 percent or greater) that you can resist any action urges that arise.

2. Record the scenario on a device, perhaps using your phone or computer. You can also read it repeatedly, if that works better for you.

3. Review the emotion-driven actions you'll resist for that exposure and the alternative actions you'll do. Watch for action urges, such as reassuring yourself, analyzing your experiences, or checking how you're feeling. If you discover you're doing something like that, the alternative action is to redirect your attention to the negative feelings and the thoughts or images that are evoking those feelings.

4. If you haven't written a *value-action statement* for this emotion practice, write one now and repeat it to yourself a few times. For example, if family is an important value to you and your guilt over a divorce is preventing you from joining activities with friends, your value-action statement might read, "In order to be the mother and friend I want to be, I will face the guilt and sadness I feel about the divorce." Repeat the value-action statement several times to motivate yourself for what is to come.

5. Find a place to practice where you won't be interrupted or distracted. Close your eyes and listen to the recording. As you listen, imagine that the recorded scenario is happening now. FACE the feelings that arise the way you've learned and resist any urges to distract yourself from the experience that the visualization is triggering. Once you've anchored to your breath, open your attention to include the negative feeling. Observe your negative feelings without judging or analyzing them. Stay with the feelings and watch them in the moment.

6. Repeat step 5 until your discomfort decreases to 50 percent or less of the maximum or peak of your distress. It's essential that you repeat thought emotion exposures within a period of time, if you can, to experience the benefit. For example, listen to the recording ten times, then take a two-minute break and listen to the recording ten times more, and so on.

7. At the end of each thought emotion exposure practice session, complete the bottom half of the log. It's essential that you spend some time reflecting on what you learned from every emotion exposure you complete. Don't forget to describe what you learned that was helpful. Did what you expected to happen occur? And most important, were you able to tolerate the negative feelings?

Wrap Up

Emotion exposure builds emotion tolerance, and with greater tolerance—here's the paradox—the intensity and persistence of your emotional reactions become more reasonable and flexible. Your emotions rise and fall in a few minutes rather than persisting for hours or days. Then your emotional reactions become more stable and predictable.

In the next chapter, you'll learn skills to enhance happiness and well-being. The CBT skills that you've learned so far have focused on decreasing your distress and improving your effectiveness in life. These are great skills, but there's more to life than feeling less anxious, down, or frustrated. There's building a life worth living. Emotional well-being skills can help you do that.

CHAPTER 8

Emotional Well-Being Skills

The CBT skills that you've learned thus far are primarily focused on dampening intense *negative* emotions, such as anxiety, depression, anger, or guilt, and the problematic actions that tend to accompany them. But there's more to life than just feeling less anxious, angry, or depressed. There are the positive emotions that promote your emotional well-being and add joy to your life.

Emotional well-being skills are a set of strategies that come from the field of positive psychology (Seligman, Rashid, and Parks 2006). Emotional well-being skills are *inside skills* because they target positive thoughts and feelings and the inner strengths that promote optimal functioning in life (Keyes, Fredrickson, and Park 2012; Parks and Schueller 2014). Emotional well-being skills complement the other CBT skills you've learned in this workbook. There are many emotional well-being skills. In this chapter, you'll learn several that are easy to practice and apply.

Why Are Emotional Well-Being Skills Important?

Positive psychology researchers have identified a number of benefits of emotional well-being skills (Lyubomirsky, King, and Diener 2005):

- A relatively small change in perspective can lead to astounding shifts in well-being and quality of life. For example, focusing on what you have rather than on what you desire can increase your happiness.

- Increased happiness and well-being moderate the effects of negative emotions, such as anxiety, depression, or guilt. This translates into greater resilience in the face of the inevitable bumps of life.

- Happiness and well-being increase your chances of success because they enable you to persist, and persistence is the key to personal and professional success.

Skill: Keep a Gratitude Journal

Gratitude is an attitude. It's an attitude that encourages you to appreciate what you have rather than what you don't have. It's an attitude that encourages you to appreciate what you have *now* rather reaching for something you hope will make you happier *tomorrow*. It's an attitude that challenges the belief that you can't feel satisfied until you've satisfied every need: a new car, a new experience, or a new relationship.

Perhaps the simplest way to spend time with gratitude is to keep a gratitude journal. Keeping a gratitude journal encourages you to pay attention to the good things in life that otherwise you take for granted. It's easy to get numb to the regular sources of goodness in life, and this opens you to more anxiety and depression. Writing your thoughts has far more emotional punch than just thinking about the things for which you're grateful. Journal writing puts you in touch with your experience and creates greater meaning about life and your place in it. Follow these tips to get the most out of your gratitude journal:

- **Commit to feeling more grateful and happy.** Your wish to experience more happiness and well-being through the process of spending time with gratitude is a key element. Like most activities, your motivation to do it and benefit from it makes a big difference in the success of your gratitude journal.

- **Strive for depth rather than breadth.** Elaborate in detail for each journal entry. Depth of response is more beneficial. For example, rather than listing an item, "Glen called me this morning," try "Glen took time to call me. He's busy and he didn't seem rushed in the call. He said some nice things about me and how I'm doing. I'm so fortunate to have Glen in my life."

- **Focus on people more than on things.** Although you have many things in your life for which to feel grateful, it's gratitude for the people in your life (friends, children, spouse, family members) that has the greatest influence on your happiness. Each day, enter into your journal one of the people for whom you're grateful to have in your life.

- **Include surprises.** Record events that you didn't expect, such as a call from a friend or the rosebud that just bloomed. Surprises elicit wonder and stronger feelings of gratitude.

- **Don't make it a job.** Writing once or twice per week is more helpful than journaling every day, perhaps because rigid and excessive journaling becomes drudgery. Instead, try for a few times per week. It doesn't matter when in the day you do it as long as you do it.

After a few weeks of keeping your gratitude journal, check in with yourself. Describe how you felt. Did you feel a bit lighter or less anxious? Did you smile when you entered something in your journal? Did you remember similar kindnesses from others? Did it make you want to express appreciation to others? Not just friends and family members but toward strangers on the street?

_____

_____

_____

_____

_____

_____

Skill: Send Thank You Notes

Positive relationships are one of the best predictors of happiness and well-being. Appreciating the people in your life nurtures these relationships and strong positive relationships are a primary source of happiness. You likely have people in your life whom you cherish and appreciate, but you don't always take the time to spell out the reasons why. Furthermore, you might have people from your past who have positively impacted your life, yet they have no idea.

In this skill, you'll use the Send Thank You Notes Worksheet, to identify a person for whom you're grateful, and tell them how they've impacted your life in a thank you note. As you write the note, open yourself to feelings of appreciation and happiness. Your eyes may fill with tears as you connect with a special kindness the person extended to you.

Instructions

1. Think of people who have had a positive impact on your life or who have done something generous or special for you. It could be a parent, friend, teacher, partner, or just about anyone. Try to identify someone whom you're able to visit. In the worksheet, write their names and then list the good deeds and special qualities that have brought joy and meaning into your life.

2. Write a thank you note to the person telling them how they've impacted your life for the better. Tell them how they've helped you or why you're grateful for them.

3. If possible, deliver the note in person. Read the note to them, and then allow the conversation to move forward naturally. Allow them to keep the note as a gift. If it isn't possible to meet in person, call the person and read the note over the phone, then mail it to them to keep.

Send Thank You Notes Worksheet

Name of Person	Good Deeds and Special Qualities

Describe how you felt as you wrote several thank you notes. Did you experience the feelings of appreciation again? As you wrote the note, did you remember other special people you wish to thank?

_____

_____

_____

_____

_____

_____

_____

_____

Skill: Send Mental Thank You Notes

Even if you don't send real thank you notes, you can send mental ones throughout the day. When you pass someone on the street, smile at them and then thank them silently for having brought something meaningful or fun into your life, such as "Thank you for wearing that beautiful scarf. It brightens my day." When you see the mail delivery person across the street, wave and then send a mental thank you, such as "Thank you for delivering the cards and letters that connect me to my friends and family." Keep your eyes open throughout the day for reasons to say thank you. Make a conscious effort to notice when people do good things, whether for you or for others. In your mind, thank the person for their good deed, such as "Thank you for stopping so that I can walk safely across the street."

Similarly, think of friends, coworkers, and family members to whom you would like to send mental thank you notes. Each day, set aside five minutes, close your eyes, and send mental thank you notes their way. Welcome the good feelings that come with appreciating the people in your life who cherish and appreciate you.

Skill: Savor a Memory

Savoring means being aware of pleasure and purposefully paying attention to the experience of pleasure (Bryant and Veroff 2007). Savoring encourages you to experience every aspect of pleasure: physical, sensory, emotional, and social (Bryant, Smart, and King 2005). You can savor the pleasure of the aroma and taste of a warm chocolate chip cookie, or the pleasure of a hot shower on a cold morning, or the pleasure of a sunset.

You can savor memories too, particularly memories of feeling happy, comfortable, or successful. For example, you might feel excited and happy as you remember the time you and your team won a softball game, or as you remember feeling warm and safe under the blankets at night. Savoring a memory works best when you try to remember everything about it: where you were and when it happened, who you were with, and what you were feeling and thinking.

Instructions
To savor a memory, use the Savor a Memory Worksheet.

Savor a Memory Worksheet

List three good times you had recently (e.g., favorite activities, favorite places you've visited, good times you've shared with friends or family, successes in your life):

Now, pick one of the good times from the list above and picture it in your mind. Then, write the elements of the story in the spaces below:

Describe where you were and what was happening. What did you hear, smell, see?	
Describe the good feelings you felt (e.g., happy, proud, satisfied, joyful, loved).	
Describe the thoughts going through your mind when feeling the good feelings.	
Describe your role in making this good time happen. Did you set it up or help?	
Imagine this good time leads to more good times and good feelings.	

Now that you've created a story about your good time and good feelings, read through it again. Finally, close your eyes and savor your good time by replaying your story in your mind.

Rate the intensity of the image and the good feeling on the scale below (1 = lowest intensity and 5 = highest intensity):

Intensity of Image	1	2	3	4	5
Intensity of Good Feeling	1	2	3	4	5

Practice savoring mindfully several times during the day, such as when you awaken in the morning, during lunch, and before bed. If you like, write other stories of fond memories and place them nearby to savor when a story gets a bit stale.

Skill: Meditate on Gratitude

Another way to spend time with gratitude is to make a gratitude meditation and listen to it daily. Gratitude happens in the present moment, and meditation, as you've learned, involves focusing on the present moment without judgment. Although people often focus on a word or phrase (such as "peace"), it's also possible to focus on what you're grateful for (the smile of your child, a favorite song, the embrace of a loved one).

Instructions

1. Find a safe, quiet place where no one is likely to disturb you. Sit or lie down in a comfortable place.

2. Make sure you're warm enough. Loosen any restrictive clothing so that you can breathe comfortably.

3. You may wish to read aloud the script below and record it so that you can play the recording while you meditate on gratitude. Try to make a recording that's about ten minutes long. Here's an example of a gratitude meditation script, but feel free to write your own if you prefer:

Close your eyes and take a slow, deep breath to bring yourself to the present moment and begin the process of feeling more peaceful and centered. Breathe into the belly so it expands as you breathe in and gets smaller as you breathe out.

Take a minute or two to mentally scan your body for any areas where there is tightness, tension, or soreness. Breathe your warm, oxygen-filled breath into that area. As you breathe out, release the tension.

Notice any anxiety or sadness or other feelings, such as irritation, jealousy, or guilt. Just breathe into those emotions, noting them, and allowing them to flow out as you slowly exhale [pause for thirty seconds].

Now, with a calm body and clear mind, focus on the events, experiences, people, pets, or possessions for which you feel grateful [pause for fifteen seconds]. Recall these special gifts:

- *The gift of life itself, the most precious gift. Someone gave birth to you. Someone fed you as an infant, changed your diaper, clothed you, bathed you, taught you to speak and to understand.*

- *The gift of hearing so that you can hear and learn, whether it's the song of a bird, the notes of an orchestra, the voices of family and friends, the sound of your own breath flowing in and flowing out.*

- *The gift of a heartbeat: steady, regular, moment after moment, pumping fresh, life-giving blood to all your organs.*

[Pause for thirty seconds.]

Now think about all the things we have today that make your life easier and more comfortable than life was for your great-grandparents:

- *You flip a switch and light appears.*

- *You turn a tap and clean, drinkable water flows.*

- *You adjust a thermostat and a room grows warmer or cooler.*

- *You have a roof to keep you dry when it rains, walls to keep out the cold wind, windows to let in the light, screens to keep out insects.*

- *You enter a vehicle and it takes you where you wish to go.*

- *You have access to machines that wash your clothes. And you have clothes to wear and places to store them.*

- *There are machines that store your food at the right temperature and help you cook it.*

- *You have indoor plumbing.*

- *You have public libraries with thousands of books, free for anyone to borrow and read.*

- *You have public schools where you learned to read and write, skills that were available to very few just a few hundred years ago.*

[Pause for thirty seconds.]

Now, take a moment to reflect on all the thousands of people who have worked hard, many without knowing you at all, to make your life easier or more pleasant:

- *People who plant, grow, and harvest your food.*

- *People who transport that food to market.*

- *People who make the roads and railways easier to transport the food.*

- *People who maintain, drive, load, and unload those vehicles.*

- *People who designed the store, the shelves, the packaging that keeps the food safe and allows you to find what you want.*

- *Postal workers who sort the mail. Others who deliver it.*

- *People who maintain the servers so you can get and send email and access the internet.*

- *People who gather, sort, and dispose of trash and recycling to keep your home and communities clean and safe.*

- *People who gather news stories and photos to keep you informed and amused.*

- *People who play sports or create art or music that entertains and enriches you.*

[Pause for thirty seconds.]

Now, consider the people and pets you know who enrich your life. Those who smile at you and cheer you on. Those family, friends, acquaintances, colleagues, and peers. Those ancestors who worked so you could live well. Those friends who support you when you need a shoulder to cry on or a helping hand [pause for thirty seconds].

Now, take a moment to reflect on your own reasons for feeling grateful in this moment. There is so much to feel grateful for in this moment now. Gratitude fills your heart and mind, uplifting your spirit [pause for thirty seconds].

When you finish the meditation, rest quietly for several minutes. Notice how you feel throughout your body. Notice your emotions and thoughts now as compared to before you meditated. Do not judge, just notice. Then, gently stretch your hands and arms, feet and legs. If you choose to stand, do so slowly.

Describe how you felt as you read, recorded, and then listened to the gratitude meditation. Did you experience feelings of happiness or peace, a sense of well-being? Did you feel less worried and stressed? Did you feel a bit more hopeful about your future and a little less down?

_____

_____

_____

_____

_____

_____

_____

Skill: Cultivate Kindness

Small acts of kindness toward others not only help them but it also helps you. Performing small acts of kindness boosts your happiness and connection to others. Acts of kindness can include altruistic activities such as volunteering, caring for a friend or coworker during a tough time, or reaching out to a stranger in need.

Smaller acts of kindness can increase your happiness too, and because they're small, you can do them every day. The key to small acts of kindness is to go beyond your regular level of kindness. If you already hold doors open for people, holding open another door probably won't boost your happiness all that much.

Instructions

1. Look at the list on the Small Acts of Kindness Worksheet. Circle those you'd like to try.

2. Watch other people and note their small acts of kindness and add these to the list as well. At first, it might be difficult to identify opportunities for small acts of kindness, but as you practice and pay attention, you'll notice other opportunities to cultivate kindness.

3. Set yourself a goal of performing one small act of kindness each day for a week. Work toward three acts of kindness every day over the next few weeks.

Small Acts of Kindness Worksheet

Buy a cup of coffee for a stranger.	Take a neighbor's trash cans to the street for pickup.	Offer directions to someone who looks lost.
Pick up trash from the street.	Give a friend a ride to the airport.	Help someone carry groceries to their car.
Leave a larger than usual tip for service.	Write a nice compliment on the dinner check.	Offer to wash your neighbor's car when you wash yours.
Offer to photocopy for a coworker.	Offer to walk your friend's dog for them.	Bring donuts to the office for coworkers.
Pay for the coffee for the person behind you in line.	Share your umbrella with a stranger on a rainy day.	Invite someone to exit a doorway before you.
Share flowers from your garden with coworkers.	Rake leaves out of the gutter in your neighborhood.	Send art supplies to a local elementary school.

Describe how you felt as you brainstormed ideas for small acts of kindness. Did you experience feelings of kindness? Did you feel good feelings toward others?

_____

_____

_____

_____

Skill: Develop Meaning and Purpose

Having a sense of meaning and purpose associated with the past, present, and future can improve well-being. You can develop a sense of meaning and purpose through writing a story about your life.

Instructions

1. Write one to two pages about your past. Describe how you overcame significant challenges using your strengths. Give yourself an hour or two to write, wait a few days, and then come back and review what you wrote. Feel free to make revisions.

2. Next, write one to two pages about who you are now. Describe how your present self is different from your past self. Include the ways you've grown and the strengths you've developed.

3. Finally, write one to two pages about your imagined future self. What kind of person do you hope to become? How will your strengths grow? What would you like to achieve? Then, describe how you can go about achieving these things.

4. Save your story and review it regularly. Update the story as you grow.

Skill: Imagine Your Ideal Self

Imagining your ideal self in the future generates feelings of joy and excitement in the present for your future self. This skill is a catalyst for change too. Imagining your ideal self in the future can motivate you to act toward achieving the life that person will want to live (Sheldon and Lyubomirsky 2006).

Instructions

1. Find a safe, quiet place where no one is likely to disturb you. Sit or lie down in a comfortable place.

2. Imagine yourself in the future, living the life you've dreamt of with all the people you want to share it with. Imagine that you achieved everything that you're struggling for now and you're proud of your achievements.

3. Immerse yourself in this imagined self. Open yourself to the happiness and positive feelings that you think you will feel in the future.

Now, consider the specific actions you can take to achieve that stage of life. Describe these actions.

_____

_____

_____

_____

_____

_____

Skill: Compliment Yourself

Who doesn't feel a sense of pride and pleasure when someone compliments them? Compliments redirect our attention to the positive aspects of ourselves. Compliments also encourage us to act positively. You can feel pride and contentment when you actively compliment yourself on the qualities others admire in you. You'll use the Positive Qualities Assessment Worksheet to practice this skill.

Instructions

1. Using the worksheet, list the positive qualities that you appreciate about yourself. Consider your *physical* qualities, such as the color of your eyes or your smile. Consider your *temperamental* qualities, such as your patience or good humor. Last, consider your *relational* qualities, such as your steadfastness as a friend or kindness toward strangers. If it's difficult for you to identify qualities about yourself that you admire, consider what others have told you that they admire about you.

2. Find a safe, quiet place where no one is likely to disturb you. Sit or lie down in a comfortable place. Close your eyes and take three slow deep breaths.

3. Think through the list of positive qualities and repeat to yourself, for example:

   - I like that I'm patient and compassionate toward others.

   - I like that I am a good listener.

   - I like that I'm a good artist.

4. After five minutes, open yourself to the warm feelings that come with appreciating yourself for who you are now.

5. In order to carry these good feelings into your day, select a positive quality about yourself that you appreciate and go through the day wearing it like your favorite sweater. For example, walk through the day wearing "I like that I'm patient and compassionate toward others."

Positive Qualities Assessment Worksheet		
Physical Qualities	Temperamental Qualities	Relational Qualities

Now reflect on what it was like to wear the positive qualities throughout the day. Did you feel happier with yourself? Did you notice that you acted in a way that others appreciated? Did you find yourself thinking about other qualities that you admire about yourself? Describe your experiences.

_____

_____

_____

_____

Skill: Design a Beautiful Day

Perhaps you've had a moment when you smile, nod your head in contentment, and say to yourself, "What a beautiful day." Beautiful days can affect us like that. In this skill, you'll design a beautiful day in the future and plan how you can make the day as close to perfect as possible. This skill pays off twice: as you design the beautiful day and as you live it. Use the Design a Beautiful Day Worksheet to describe the day in as much detail as possible.

Instructions

1. Take a few minutes and consider what makes a beautiful day for you. Describe the day in as much detail as possible. Strive to involve others in your beautiful day. This doesn't mean you can't have any alone time, but try not to spend the entire day alone.

2. Include little details in your beautiful day. Want to splurge on a donut on a weekday morning? Write it down. Want to stretch in the sunshine at lunch? Write it down. However, don't plan your beautiful day so much that you lose the joy of spontaneous moments.

3. Break routine and do something new on your beautiful day. It doesn't have to be expensive or a big production, just different. For example, get up a little earlier than usual and enjoy your coffee on the deck. Write it down.

4. When you finally have your beautiful day, accept that it won't be exactly as you planned it. Accept the twists and turns as they come, and savor them. Mindfully appreciate the beautiful day. Live each moment of the day and appreciate it with all your senses.

Design a Beautiful Day Worksheet

Skill: Forgive to Live Free

Holding on to past resentments drains joy and meaning from the present moment and takes you back to the anger and disappointment of the past all over again. To forgive is to decide to let go of resentment toward the person who hurt you. By forgiving, you're accepting what happened and finding a way to live with it. Forgiveness doesn't happen overnight, and it's not easy to do. Forgiveness takes time, and for most people, it's a gradual process that happens in the present moment. Use the Forgive to Live Free Worksheet to help practice this skill.

Instructions

1. List the people and the incidents from your past that you wish to forgive. Beside each name, describe how the negative encounter hurt you. Try to name all the feelings you experienced then, such as sad, angry, disappointed, heartbroken, or betrayed. As you describe the hurtful encounters, notice how those same feelings arise again.

2. Close your eyes, take two slow, deep breaths, and relax for a few minutes. Next, imagine each name on the list, and in your heart, say to yourself, "I forgive you." Repeat the phrase under your breath as you slowly exhale.

3. Relax into the lightness of forgiveness. Breathe slowly and deeply for several minutes.

4. Open your eyes and over each name and incident on the worksheet, write in bold, "FORGIVEN" and "FREE TO LIVE."

Forgive to Live Free Worksheet	
Name of Person	Hurtful Incident

Wrap Up

Feeling better is not the same as feeling happy. The emotional well-being skills in this chapter complement the other CBT skills you've learned in this workbook. Emotional well-being skills don't focus on decreasing negative emotions. Rather, they focus on increasing positive emotions, such as happiness and a sense of well-being. Furthermore, these skills build a strong foundation of joy, meaning, and appreciation for yourself and others that insulates you from the inevitable ups and downs of life.

In the final chapter, you'll put together a plan to practice regularly what you've learned. With practice, your comfort and confidence in the skills in this workbook will strengthen and deepen. A solid and clear practice plan will help you get the most from the life-changing CBT skills you've learned.

CHAPTER 9

Put It All Together

With practice, your comfort and confidence with the skills you've learned will strengthen and deepen. In this final chapter, you'll put it all together to build a practice plan to do just that. A plan will help you see the path forward. It's not as overwhelming as it may seem. Just fifteen minutes each day of focused practice can make a huge difference in your confidence with the skills. With more confidence comes less resistance to applying the skills in the moment, which is what change is all about.

At the same time, many of the workbook skills are more difficult to apply when you're in the thick of it, that is, when you're feeling anxious, sad, angry, or upset. In this chapter, you'll learn an approach to build your confidence so you can apply the skills when it counts: when you're feeling what you're feeling.

Build Your Practice Plan

You'll create your practice plan from a menu of CBT that you'll practice in two ways:

- **Daily practice.** Many CBT skills can be practiced daily, such as 4-7-8 breathing or progressive muscle relaxation. These practices will take five to fifteen minutes depending on the skill. Try to practice these skills at the same time each day, which will help you remember to practice. If possible, practice in the same environment, such as in your bedroom. Select a period during the day when you can be alone and you're not likely to be interrupted. It could be before lunch at work or before bed. Think of each practice as an appointment with yourself. The more often you show up, the more benefit you'll get from the skills over time.

- **Situational or event practice.** You'll practice certain CBT skills relative to events or situations as they arise in your personal and work life, like assertiveness or using I-messages. Some events may arise daily, weekly, or monthly.

Each component of your practice plan will strengthen one or more core CBT skills. There are in-the-moment skills that can relax your mind and body and create a calm physical foundation to practice and apply the other skills. Your practice plan will include emotion exposure skills to strengthen your emotion tolerance in general as well as practical skills such as problem-solving and breaking down tasks that you'll apply as they arise in specific situations. Use the CBT Skills Worksheet to determine which skills work best for you.

Instructions

1. Review the CBT skills and decide which skills will be the most useful given the typical situations that arise in your life that upset you.

2. Place a check mark (✓) next to each skill that's a good fit then note the amount of time (e.g., ten minutes) and frequency (daily, weekly, monthly) you'll practice them.

CBT Skills Worksheet				
Skill	✓	Page	Time	Frequency
Chapter 1: Motivation Skills				
Set Goals				
Consider the Costs vs. Benefits of Change				
Consider the Concerns of Others				
Identify Your Values				
Develop Value-Action Statements				
Rehearse in Your Mind				
Take Another Seat				
Chapter 2: Relaxation Skills				
Breathe with Your Abdomen				
Breathe Four Square				
Breathe 4-7-8				
Relax Your Muscles Progressively				
Release-Only to Relax				
Relax on Cue				
Apply Relaxation in the Moment				
Release Tension Quickly				
Relax and Refresh				
Chapter 3: Mindfulness Skills				
Scan Your Body				
Sit in the Ring of Light				
Breathe Mindfully				
Focus on a Single Object				
Act Mindfully				

Chapter 4: Thinking Skills				
Unpack Emotional Experiences				
Record Emotional Experiences				
Evaluate Costs vs. Benefits of an Automatic Thought				
Identify Thinking Errors				
Put an Automatic Thought on Trial				
Test Automatic Thoughts with Experiments				
Look Through the Lens of Time				
Chapter 5: Interpersonal Effectiveness Skills				
Listen and Respond				
Use I-Messages				
Make Everyday Requests				
Stand Your Ground				
Build an Assertiveness Practice Ladder, Then Practice				
Bookend with Validation				
Play the Broken Record				
Agree to Disagree				
Pick the Flower and Ignore the Weeds				
Ask for Time or a Second Opinion				
Negotiate				
Chapter 6: Time and Task Management Skills				
Increase Time and Task Awareness				
Manage Time				
Practice Strategic Time Management				
Break Down Tasks				
Prioritize Tasks				
Plan Ahead				

Do It Now			
Solve Problems			
Chapter 7: Emotion Exposure Skills			
Identify Features of Negative Feelings			
Connect with Your Values			
FACE Negative Emotions			
Resist and Delay Emotion-Driven Actions			
Build a Situation Emotion Exposure Practice Menu			
Practice Situation Emotion Exposure			
Build a Thought Emotion Exposure Practice Menu			
Practice Thought Emotion Exposure			
Chapter 8: Emotional Well-Being Skills			
Keep a Gratitude Journal			
Send Thank You Notes			
Send Mental Thank You Notes			
Savor a Memory			
Meditate on Gratitude			
Cultivate Kindness			
Develop Meaning and Purpose			
Imagine Your Ideal Self			
Compliment Yourself			
Design a Beautiful Day			
Forgive to Live Free			

Practice, Practice, Practice

Now that you have a practice plan, use the CBT Skills Practice Log to track the number of times you practice these skills.

Instructions

1. Track how often you practice each skill from the CBT Skills Worksheet.

2. In the Comments column, describe what you did and what you learned that was helpful to you.

CBT Skills Practice Log

Chapter	CBT Skill	M	T	W	Th	F	Sa	S	Comments

Skill: Cognitive Rehearsal

Self-efficacy is the belief that you possess the skills and knowledge necessary to achieve a desired goal, and confidence is the strength of that belief (Bandura 1977). In this case, it's how confident you are that the CBT skills you've learned and practiced will help you meet the goals you created in chapter 1 (Motivation Skills). In particular, it's vital that you're confident you can apply the skills when you need them the most—in a moment of distress—and that the skills work then too. Cognitive rehearsal is a great CBT strategy to build that kind of confidence (Driskell, Cooper, and Moran 1994; Rice 2015). Cognitive rehearsal can increase confidence in any of the skills you've learned, whether it's breathing slowly and deeply when you're feeling anxious, or repeating a coping statement to yourself when you're feeling depressed, or breaking down a task when you're feeling overwhelmed.

Instructions

1. Select a CBT skill from the list at the beginning of this chapter. Review the skill so that you know how to do it.

2. Identify a recent event in which you were feeling upset and you think the coping skill will help. Select an event that is fresh in your mind and therefore easy to recall and visualize. Try for an event that, when you visualize it, will evoke a moderate level of distress (4 to 6 on a 10-point scale, where 10 is extreme).

3. Close your eyes and imagine the event. Imagine specific details about the situation and setting. Where are you? Who is there and what are they doing? What's happening? Bring in all your senses. What do you see, hear, smell? Notice any sensations in your body—warmth, tingling, tension—that are part of what you're feeling.

4. Rate the vividness of the image on a 10-point scale, from 0 (not at all vivid) to 10 (intensely vivid). Stay with the scene until it is very vivid (6 or above on the 10-point scale). If you can't create a vivid image, try a different event that you can recall in more detail.

5. Rate your level of confidence that the skill can help you cope with the event on a scale of 0 to 100 percent, where 100 percent is completely confident that the skill will help.

6. Rate your level of distress or emotion on the 10-point scale. Try for at least a moderate level of distress, somewhere between 4 and 6.

7. Now use the coping skill that you selected. For example, if the skill is 4-7-8 breathing, then breathe in this way. If the skill is to use a coping statement, repeat the coping statement to yourself. Continue to use the skill until the level of distress or emotion decreases at least by half. For example, if the initial level of distress is 4 to 6, continue until the level of distress is 2 to 3.

8. Return to imagining the event until you feel distressed again and then repeat steps 6 and 7.

9. Last, re-rate your level of confidence that the skill can help you cope with the event on a scale of 0 to 100 percent, where 100 percent is completely confident that the skill will help. Continue cognitive rehearsal until your confidence level is 90 percent or greater.

Describe what cognitive rehearsal was like for you and what you learned that was helpful.

_____

_____

_____

_____

_____

_____

_____

_____

Skill: Get Ahead of Distress

Cognitive rehearsal is a great way to get ahead of future upsetting or distressing events. Through cognitive rehearsal, you can establish that a particular CBT skill can help you cope effectively with an event if and when it happens. Preparing ahead in this way builds your confidence that you can get through an upsetting event, which will help you worry less about it.

Instructions

1. Follow the same cognitive rehearsal steps as above, but this time, visualize an upsetting event or situation that hasn't yet happened. As before, imagine who will be there, what's happening, and how you're feeling. Stay with the visualization until you're feeling a moderate (4 to 6) level of distress.

2. Turn your attention to the coping skill you've selected. In your mind's eye, visualize using the CBT skill. Continue to imagine using the skill until your distress level decreases by at least 50 percent.

3. If you didn't observe a significant decrease in your distress level, select a different coping skill and repeat the process. This is a great way to optimize the CBT skill for the upsetting event. This adds to your confidence that a particular skill works well in a particular situation. Continue to practice cognitive rehearsal until your confidence level is at least 80 to 90 percent.

Remember that certain CBT skills, such as assertiveness or negotiating, don't guarantee you'll get what you want, but cognitive rehearsal will help you feel less anxious or upset while you try to get it.

Wrap Up

So, you've created a practice plan that puts it all together. But now comes the most important part: committing to those fifteen minutes each day strengthening your skills and deepening the positive changes the skills will bring your way. But how do you commit to fifteen minutes of practice each day? The same way that you eat an elephant: one piece at a time, or in your case, one minute at a time. Good luck!

References

Balban, M. Y., E. Neri, M. M. Kogon, L. Weed, B. Nouriani, J. Booil, J. Holl, J. M. Zeitzer, D. Spiegel, and A. D. Huberman. 2023. Brief structured respiration practices enhance mood and reduce physiological arousal. *Cell Reports Medicine*, 4, 1–10.

Bandura, A. 1977. Self-efficacy: Toward a unifying theory of behavioral change. *Psychological Review*, 84 191–215.

Barlow, D. H., L. B. Allen, and M. L. Choate. 2016. Toward a unified treatment for emotional disorders. *Behavior Therapy*, 47, 838–853.

Beck, A. T. 1964. Thinking and depression. II. Theory and therapy. *Archives of General Psychiatry*, 10, 561–571.

————. 1970. Cognitive therapy: Nature and relation to behavior therapy. *Behavior Therapy*, 1, 184–200.

————. 1976. *Cognitive therapy and the emotional disorders*. New York: International Universities Press.

Beck, A. T., G. Emery, and R. L. Greenberg. 1985. *Anxiety disorders and phobias: A cognitive perspective*. New York: Basic Books.

Beck, A. T., A. J. Rush, B. E. Shaw, and G. Emery. 1979. *Cognitive therapy of depression*. New York: Guilford Press.

Bennett-Levy, J. 2003. Mechanisms of change in cognitive therapy: The case of automatic thought records and behavioural experiments. *Behavioural and Cognitive Psychotherapy*, 31, 261–277.

Bennett-Levy, J., G. Butler, M. J. V. Fennell, A. Hackmann, M. Mueller, and D. Westbrook, (Eds.). 2004. *The Oxford guide to behavioural experiments in cognitive therapy*. Oxford: Oxford University Press.

Braun, J. D., D. R. Strunk, K. E. Sasso, and A. A. Cooper. 2015. Therapist use of Socratic questioning predicts session-to-session symptom change in cognitive therapy for depression. *Behaviour Research and Therapy*, 70, 32–37.

Bryant, F. B., C. M. Smart, and S. P. King. 2005. Using the past to enhance the present: Boosting happiness through positive reminiscence. *Journal of Happiness Studies: An Interdisciplinary Forum on Subjective Well-Being*, 6, 227–260.

Bryant, F. B., and J. Veroff. 2007. *Savoring: A new model of positive experience.* Mahwah, NJ: Lawrence Erlbaum.

Butler, A. C., J. E. Chapman, E. M. Forman, and A. T. Beck. 2006. The empirical status of cognitive-behavioral therapy: A review of meta-analyses. *Clinical Psychology Review*, 26, 17–31.

Chambers, R., B. Chuen Yee Lo, and N. B. Allen. 2008. The impact of intensive mindfulness training on attentional control, cognitive style, and affect. *Cognitive Therapy and Research*, 32, 303–322.

Clark, M. E., and R. Hirschman. 1990. Effects of paced respiration on anxiety reduction in a clinical population. *Biofeedback and Self-Regulation*, 15, 273–284.

Doran, G. T. 1981. There's a S.M.A.R.T. way to write management's goals and objectives. *Management Review*, 70, 35–36.

Driskell, J. E., C. Cooper, and A. Moran. 1994. Does mental practice enhance performance? *Journal of Applied Psychology*, 79, 481–492.

Hannawa, A., and B. Spitzberg, (Eds.). 2015. *Communication competence.* Berlin: Walter de Grutyer.

Hargie, O. 2017. *Skilled interpersonal communication: Research, theory and practice* (6th ed.). London: Routledge.

Hayes, S. C., K. D. Strosahl, and K. G. Wilson. 2016. *Acceptance and commitment therapy: The process and practice of mindful change.* New York: Guilford Press.

Heiniger, L. E., G. I. Clark, and S. J. Egan. 2018. Perceptions of Socratic and non-Socratic presentation of information in cognitive behavior therapy. *Journal of Behavior Therapy and Experimental Psychiatry*, 58, 106–113.

Hofmann, S. G., A. Asnaani, I. J. Vonk, A. T. Sawyer, and A. Fang. 2012. The efficacy of cognitive behavioral therapy: A review of meta-analyses. *Cognitive Therapy and Research*, 36, 427–440.

Hofmann, S. G., A. T. Sawyer, A. A. Witt, and D. Oh. 2010. The effect of mindfulness-based therapy on anxiety and depression: A meta-analytic review. *Journal of Consulting and Clinical Psychology*, 78 169–183.

Jacobson, E. 1938. *Progressive relaxation.* Chicago: University of Chicago Press.

Kabat-Zinn, J. 1982. An outpatient program in behavioral medicine for chronic pain patients based on the practice of mindfulness meditation: Theoretical considerations and preliminary results. *General Hospital Psychiatry*, 4, 33–47.

———. 1990. *Full catastrophe living: Using the wisdom of your body and mind to face stress, pain, and illness.* New York: Delacourt.

Keyes, C. L., B. L. Fredrickson, and N. Park. 2012. Positive psychology and the quality of life. In K. C. Land, A. C. Michalos, and M. J. Sirgy (Eds.), *Handbook of social indications and quality of life research*. Dordrecht: Springer.

Linehan, M. 2014. *DBT Skills training manual* (2nd ed.) New York: Guilford Press.

Lyubomirsky, S., L. King, and E. Diener. 2005. The benefits of frequent positive affect: Does happiness lead to success? *Psychological Bulletin*, 131, 803–855.

McCaul, K. D., S. Solomon, and D. S. Holmes. 1979. Effects of paced respiration and expectations on physiological and psychological responses to threat. *Journal of Personality and Social Psychology*, 37, 564–571.

Moreno, J. D. 2014. *Impromptu man: J. L. Moreno and the origins of psychodrama, encounter culture, and the social network* (p. 50). New York: Bellevue Literary Press.

Müller, R., C. Peter, A. Cieza, et al. 2015. Social skills: A resource for more social support, lower depression levels, higher quality of life and participation in individuals with spinal cord injury? *Archives of Physical Medicine and Rehabilitation*, 96, 447–455.

Öst, L. G. 1987. Applied relaxation: Description of a coping technique and review of controlled studies. *Behavior Research and Therapy*, 25, 397–409.

Parks, A. C., and S. Schueller. 2014. *The Wiley Blackwell handbook of positive psychology interventions*. West Sussex, UK: John Wiley and Sons.

Rice, R. H. 2015. Cognitive-behavioral therapy. *The Sage Encyclopedia of Theory in Counseling and Psychotherapy*, 1 194.

Seligman, M. E. P., T. Rashid, and A. C. Parks. 2006. Positive psychotherapy. *American Psychologist*, 61, 774–788.

Sheldon, K. M., and S. Lyubomirsky. 2006. How to increase and sustain positive emotion: The effects of expressing gratitude and visualizing best possible selves. *The Journal of Positive Psychology*, 1, 73–82.

Tompkins, M. A. 2021. *The Anxiety and depression workbook: Simple, effective CBT techniques to manage moods and feel better now*. Oakland, CA: New Harbinger Publications.

Trousselard, M., D. Steiler, D. Claverie, and F. Canini. 2014. The history of mindfulness put to the test of current scientific data: Unresolved questions. *Encephale*, 40, 474–480.

Wasserman, T., and L. Wasserman. 2020. Motivation: State, trait, or both. In T. Wasserman and L. Wasserman (Eds.), *Motivation, effort, and the neural network model: Applications and implications* (pp. 93–102). Edinburgh: Springer, Cham.

Michael A. Tompkins, PhD, ABPP, is a board-certified psychologist in behavioral and cognitive psychology. He is codirector of the San Francisco Bay Area Center for Cognitive Therapy, and a faculty member of the Beck Institute for Cognitive Behavior Therapy. Tompkins is author or coauthor of fifteen books, and presents to national and international audiences on cognitive behavioral therapy (CBT) and related topics. His work has been highlighted by media outlets, including in *The New York Times*, *The Wall Street Journal*, on television (TLC, A&E), and on radio (KQED, NPR).

Foreword writer **Judith S. Beck, PhD,** is president of the Beck Institute for Cognitive Behavior Therapy, and clinical professor of psychology in psychiatry at the University of Pennsylvania. She is author of the seminal text, *Cognitive Behavior Therapy*, which has been translated into more than twenty languages, and whose third edition contains a recovery orientation.

Real change *is* possible

For more than forty-five years, New Harbinger has published proven-effective self-help books and pioneering workbooks to help readers of all ages and backgrounds improve mental health and well-being, and achieve lasting personal growth. In addition, our spirituality books offer profound guidance for deepening awareness and cultivating healing, self-discovery, and fulfillment.

Founded by psychologist Matthew McKay and Patrick Fanning, New Harbinger is proud to be an independent, employee-owned company. Our books reflect our core values of integrity, innovation, commitment, sustainability, compassion, and trust. Written by leaders in the field and recommended by therapists worldwide, New Harbinger books are practical, accessible, and provide real tools for real change.

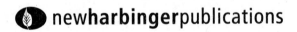 **newharbinger**publications

MORE BOOKS from
NEW HARBINGER PUBLICATIONS

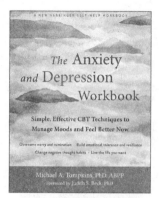
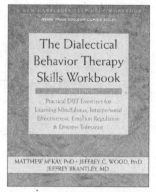
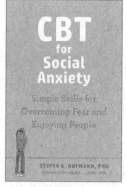
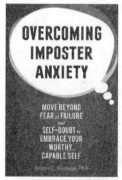
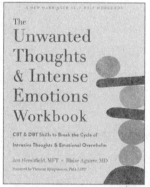
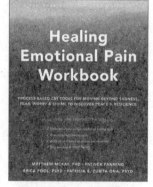

Did you know there are **free tools** you can download for this book?

Free tools are things like **worksheets**, **guided meditation exercises**, and **more** that will help you get the most out of your book.

You can download free tools for this book—whether you bought or borrowed it, in any format, from any source—from the New Harbinger website. All you need is a NewHarbinger.com account. Just use the URL provided in this book to view the free tools that are available for it. Then, click on the "download" button for the free tool you want, and follow the prompts that appear to log in to your NewHarbinger.com account and download the material.

You can also save the free tools for this book to your **Free Tools Library** so you can access them again anytime, just by logging in to your account! Just look for this button on the book's free tools page.

+ Save this to my free tools library

If you need help accessing or downloading free tools, visit **newharbinger.com/faq** or contact us at **customerservice@newharbinger.com**.